The 30 Day Vegan Whole Foods Challenge

The Essential Beginner`s Guide to Great Food, Good Health, and Easy Weight Loss;

With 60 Compliant, Simple, and Delicious Vegan Recipes

AUTHOR: JESSICA TROYER

Legal & Disclaimer

The information contained in this book and its contents is not designed to replace or take the place of any form of medical or professional advice; and is not meant to replace the need for independent medical, financial, legal or other professional advice or services, as may be required. The content and information in this book have been provided for educational and entertainment purposes only.

The content and information contained in this book have been compiled from sources deemed reliable, and it is accurate to the best of the Author's knowledge, information, and belief. However, the Author cannot guarantee its accuracy and validity and cannot be held liable for any errors and omissions. Further, changes are periodically made to this book as and when needed. Where appropriate and necessary, you must consult a professional (including but not limited to your doctor, attorney, financial advisor or such other professional advisor) before using any of the suggested remedies, techniques, or information in this book.

Upon using the contents and information contained in this book, you agree to hold harmless the Author from and against any damages, costs, and expenses, including any legal fees potentially resulting from the application of any of the information provided by this book. This disclaimer applies to any loss, damages or injury caused by the use and application, whether directly or indirectly, of any advice or information presented, whether for breach of contract, tort, negligence, personal injury, criminal intent, or under any other cause of action.

You agree to accept all risks of using the information presented in this book.

You agree that by continuing to read this book, where appropriate and necessary, you shall consult a professional (including but not limited to your doctor, attorney, or financial advisor or such other advisor as needed) before using any of the suggested remedies, techniques, or information in this book.

All product names, trademarks and registered trademarks are property of their respective owners. All company, product and service names used in this book are for identification purposes only. Use of these names, trademarks and brands does not imply endorsement.

Contents

Introduction

Let me start your journey by thanking you and expressing my utmost gratitude and appreciation to you and your kind gesture for taking the time to purchase this book.

While writing this book, my aim was to ensure that readers of all experience levels were able to easily grasp the concept of both Veganism and Whole Foods Diet! And in doing so, I tried my very best to keep this book as accessible and easy to understand as possible.

The whole book has been divided into individual chapters, which are themselves divided into bite-sized sections, each of which focuses on a single topic.

While reading the book, you will notice that the first part of the book fully focuses on explaining the ins and outs of Whole Foods Diet, while the second one focuses on teaching you the fundamentals of Veganism.

Once you are done with the intro chapters, you will find a plethora of amazing Whole Foods recipes that will fully comply with your Vegan lifestyle!

I hope you enjoy the book and fully live out the Whole Foods diet while following your Vegan lifestyle!

Part 1: The Fundamentals of the Whole Foods Diet

As mentioned in the introduction, the first part of this book is about making yourself comfortable by helping you wrap the concept of the Whole Foods Diet around your head.

Throughout this part, you will find information covering topics such as:

- The basic definition of the Whole Foods Diet
- The different food groups and the standards of food you should try to pursue
- The food groups that make you unhealthier
- The restrictions of the diet and the food groups you are allowed to eat and the ones you are required to get rid of.
- What you should do after your 30-day Whole Foods challenge is complete
- How to prepare your kitchen by having the most crucial components for a better experience
- The side effects you should be aware of
- How you can successfully carry out your Whole Foods journey
- The advantages of following a Whole Foods Diet

Chapter 1: What Exactly is a Whole Foods Diet?

Considering the recent statistics, more than 10,000 people all around the world have already jumped into the Whole Foods Diet bandwagon and are already sharing their "Life Changing" experiences.

So, naturally, the first question that pops to mind is obviously the most basic one.

"What exactly is a Whole Foods diet?"

Whole Foods diet is a month-long (30 days) program that encourages an individual to get rid of some specific food groups to purify or "Cleanse" the whole ecosystem of the body.

This particular diet promises to bless an individual with a large array of benefits that are both physical and psychological.

This systemic reset will seamlessly allow your body to re-invigorate the metabolic, digestive, and defensive mechanism of the body and in turn, make the whole body much healthier overall.

The 30 Day Whole Foods Challenge program tries to fully "RESET" the whole metabolic system of the body and completely reshape how you interact with your food on a daily basis.

Generally speaking, the menu of a Whole Foods diet very closely resembles that of a Paleo Diet, which promotes a high protein and low carb diet.

But the Whole Foods Diet is much more advanced and strict regarding elimination. Unlike Paleo, there's no option to cheat here. For one whole month, you are required to get rid of your indulgences.

Food groups such as inflammatory groups such as grains, dairy, sugar, alcohols, and legumes are required to be completely eliminated.

Not to mention, junk foods such as Burgers or even Pizza are off the table as well.

The restrictions of the diet should not be regarded as a limiting factor to your lifestyle, but a means through which you will be able to re-orient your food habits so that you can enjoy cleaner and simpler foods.

As much difficult as the whole journey may sound like, I will try my very best to provide you with the guidelines required to make your journey as smooth as possible.

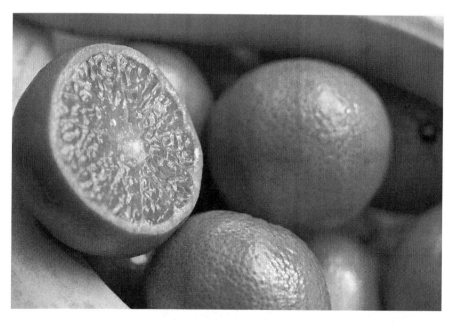

Chapter 2: Why Should You Follow a Whole Foods Diet?

You must be wondering now, why should you follow a Whole Foods diet right? I mean, in the first chapter I have already talked a bit about how thousands of people are already in the Whole Foods cycle, but I didn't talk about the benefits, right?

While the list of benefits that can be achieved through a proper Whole Foods reset would easily fill up even the largest bucket, I am going to list out some of the more prominent ones here that are bound to encourage you for a better future.

Improved skin, nails, and hair condition: Let's start with one of the most unexpected benefits first! Once you start to cut down the unhealthy foods from your body, the condition of your skin and nails will start to improve.

More available energy to spend: It has been seen that people who are on a Whole Foods diet tend to have about three times more energy than a person who isn't. This is primarily because you are fueling up your body with a 100% pure green energy.

However, it should be noted that the energy won't necessarily be instantaneous. You will feel a little bit of sluggishness during the first week or so, but once your body adjusts itself to the changed diet, you soon feel the surge of energy flowing through your veins.

Will help you trim down excess weight: Since you are completely getting rid of sugar alongside any junk foods! The Whole Foods Diet will have a huge impact eventually when it comes to trimming down your fat. Through Whole Foods Diet, you are promoting your mind to pay more attention to the food that you are eating, thus eliminating more fatty foods from your list, which will, in turn, cause your body to eventually lose weight and attain the physique that you have been dreaming of! If you just do a little research, you are bound to find thousands of stories of man and women successfully losing their weight through Whole Foods diet.

It will improve your sleeping condition: The Whole Foods Diet actually goes a long way when it comes to improving and regulating the hormones in your body. This will help you improve how your body manages its internal sleep timer and improve your sleeping patterns.

It will help you stay focused all day: When you are gathering your food from quality resources, it will keep pumping you up with energy at a slow, yet steady rate. This will keep you healthy and energized all throughout the day.

The diet will break any sentimental attachment you may have with food: Emotions tend to control the type of food that you swallow more often than you might think. If you are feeling sad, then you will soon go for a chocolate milkshake! If you are happy, then you might go for something more invigorating like a pancake donut!

The Whole Foods Diet will help you make more logical decisions and help you control your food intake.

It will make you more sexually active and fertile: Too much sugar causes lots of problems, including body inflammation.

Since a Whole Foods diet will reduce the sugar intake, it will help you lower down the symptoms of diseases such as endometriosis (a disease that affects female sex organs).

This, in turn, will improve your fertility and make you feel more sexually active.

It will help you tackle Anxiety and Depression: Depression is a very common problem these days, and a more balanced link between your brain and food intake will improve the condition.

It will help you reverse serious disease symptoms: Multiple diseases such as diabetes, cerebral palsy or even multiple sclerosis can be dealt with while being on a Whole Foods diet. Patients with such diseases have shown great improvement from these chronic diseases while on a Whole Foods diet.

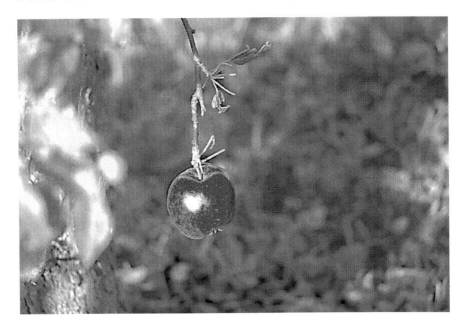

Chapter 3: Understanding Your Food

As mentioned earlier, the success of your 30 Day Whole Foods Challenge will depend on how well you are able to eliminate the unhealthy food from your life.

When looking at the dietary routine below, you should again keep in mind that there are certain items such "Eggs" or "Seafood" that are allowed in the Whole Foods diet but are restricted by the Vegan diet.

The following is yet again a generalize food list for Whole Foods dieticians; you are to ignore anything that goes against your Vegan routine.

The ingredients and recipes that are chosen for the Whole Foods Diet rely on four principles that assess the standard of the food that you are eating.

In short, foods that satisfy these four principles are the good ones!

- The food should promote a healthy psychological response from your body
- The food should promote a healthy hormonal response
- The food should improve the quality of your gut
- The food should improve your immune function and minimize your inflammation

Based on those standards, the food groups that you are allowed to use on the 30 Day Whole Foods Challenge include:

Vegetables: Don't compromise on vegetables! Including potatoes as well! There's no restriction here.

Fruits: It should be noted that fruits are allowed in moderation in a Whole Foods diet as they are sugar machines.

Unprocessed Meats: Always go for unprocessed meats as processed foods tend to add sugar and other preservatives. However, Sausage works. *Warning! Not allowed in Vegan Diet!*

Seafood: Fish and Shellfish are allowed on a Whole Foods diet. *Warning! Not allowed in Vegan Diet!*

Eggs: Eggs should be on your breakfast list as well. *Warning! Not allowed in Vegan Diet!*

Nuts and Seeds: All nuts are fully allowed during your 30 Day Whole Foods Challenge except peanuts (as they are legumes).

Oil and Ghee: You can go for unprocessed extra virgin olive oil and unprocessed extra virgin coconut oil and Ghee.

Coffee: This should come as a great joy to coffee lovers! While you are on the 30 Day Whole Foods Challenge, you are allowed to go for coffee. Just make sure you don't add any milk products or sugar. You may use almond milk though

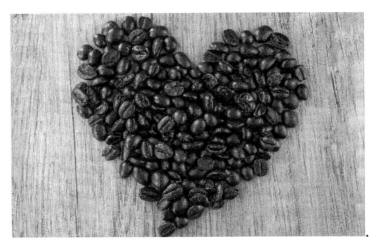

That being said, the following food groups are completely restricted:

Dairy: This means that you are not allowed to go for cow milk, cheese, cream, yogurt, sour cream, butter or even kefir. Only ghee is an exception.

Grains: Such as corns, rice, wheat, quinoa, millet, amaranth, sorghum, buckwheat, sprouted grains, and Bulgur are off the table.

Alcohol: This might come as a little bit harsh, but alcohol is completely restricted to the 30-Day Whole Foods Challenge, either for drinking or cooking.

Legumes: Legumes such as soy sauce, tofu, peanuts, and lentils are off the table as well.

Extra Sugar: Any added sugars (even artificial sweeteners) are to be avoided. Honey, agave, maple syrup, Stevia are all off the table.

Carrageenan, Sulfites, or MSG: Try to avoid processed foods.

Any "Junk" Food: Junk and baked foods are prohibited during a 30 Day Whole Foods Challenge, even if they are made using Whole Foods Diet compliant ingredients.

As an exception though, you can have:

- Fruit juice
- Green beans, sugar snap peas, and snow peas
- Vinegar

The Whole Foods Diet is completely designed around all of these food groups in order to target and improve specific parts of our health.

To break them down, these include:

Breaking an unhealthy relationship with food: The Whole Foods Diet will help you clear up any psychological or emotional relation that you might have with unhealthy food. By eliminating nutrient, poor, calorie dense food that promotes overconsumption.

Improve metabolism: The meal plan and regulation that are offered by the Whole Foods Diet will help you restore your hormonal levels and regulate the blood sugar. Over time, this will help your body to use fat as a fuel. As a result, your energy levels will increase, and you will trim a bit of fat in the process as well.

Improve digestive system: The gut will be helped by your Whole Foods program as foods that often prevent the gut from working properly are completely eliminated from the diet. This gives your gut time to heal and calm down your immune system in the process.

Soothe and calm an over-reactive Immune System: The Whole Foods Diet is really an Anti-Inflammatory diet that helps to calm down an over-reactive immune system. Various symptoms such as aches and pains are relieved during this diet.

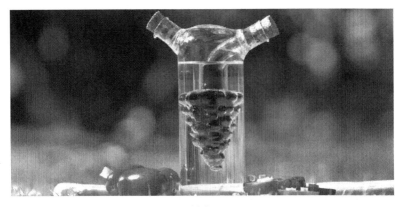

Chapter 4: Preparing Your Kitchen for the Journey

Before diving into the recipes, it is essential that you know about the utensils that you are going to need in order to properly prepare the meals ahead.

I am pretty sure that you already have the following items in your kitchen, but if you are a complete beginner! Then this brief chapter will help you out a lot.

Don't stress too much though! Just relax and try to keep things handy.

Saucepan: 1-2 quarts of small saucepan

Dutch oven: 3-4-quart Dutch oven for large dishes

Frying Pans: Frying pans (skillets)

Sauté Pan: High-walled Sauté pans should be on your list as well.

Strainer: Strainer for allowing you to drain water from boiled vegetables or broth, which can also be used as a steamer rack with large sized stock pot

Measuring cups and spoons: A set of measuring cups and spoons, keep larger sized glass measuring cup as well

Baking Sheet: Baking sheets that will be required for roasting vegetables or meat

Cutting Board: A nice cutting board as you will be doing a lot of chopping. If possible, a wooden or bamboo surfaced one as they leave less bacterial residue

Knives: Try to go for some high-quality knives. A paring knife, an 8-inch chef's knife, and a long slicing knife should be on the top of your list.

Food Processor: A food processor might sound like an expensive tool, but you will find some good fits within your budget. You should keep one handy as they will very easily help you chop up or shred ingredients to a fine consistency.

Parchment Paper: Parchment paper for lining up your baking sheets and dishes. This is much better than aluminum foil as it keeps your dishes cleaner

Garlic Press: Mincing garlic might just become one of your most hated tasks during your culinary adventures. A Garlic Press will help you mince your garlic in seconds.

Julienne Peeler: This will help you create amazing vegetable noodles that will add a hefty dose of variety to your Julienne Peeler.

Citrus Juicer: This will help you squeeze lemon and lime seamlessly.

Zester: Some recipes in this book might call require you to use zest. A zester will easily create tiny pieces orange or lemon peels for your meal.

Chapter 5: After the 30 days

So, you are done with your Whole Foods challenge, right? Imagining what you should do now?

Well, fear not!

According to the guidelines of a Whole Foods diet, there are actually 3 more steps that you should keep in consideration to the fully enjoy the benefits of a Whole Foods diet. In this chapter, we will be talking about the different steps individually.

Let's start off with the 2nd step first.

Step 2: The Step of Reintroduction

The second step, simply known as "Reintroduction" is a very crucial part of a Whole Foods journey.

Once you are done with step 1 (The Whole Foods Challenge), the next step is to simply make up a meal plan for the next 10 days, where you are going to re-introduce some of the food that you have been avoiding for the past month.

Throughout this gradual introduction, you will get the chance to properly assess how these foods are now reacting to your metabolic levels and evaluate, which ones are going to help you maintain a healthy body overall.

The plan of re-introduction will usually require you to re-introduce one food group at a time, to ensure that you are still heavily relying on your Whole Foods diet.

You can think of this stage as somewhat of a scientific trial that you are running to check if any of those previously canceled food group are worth bringing back.

This means that you are not to combine multiple major food groups. For example, you can have a slice of toasted bread with peanut butter! Rather, you should either go for bread or peanut butter.

Regardless of what you do, pay very close attention to how your body reacts and be the best judge of yourself.

A sample schedule for 10 days might include:

Day 1: You may start off by trying to re-introduce legumes and evaluate how they work.

Day 5: After a 4 days trial run, select the legumes that you want to keep and move on to re-introducing Non-Gluten grains such as corn tortilla chips or white rice.

Day 10: Finally, you should evaluate Gluten-Containing Grains to see how they react to your body.

It should be noted that throughout all of these process, you are to stick to your usual Whole Foods diet while only including the experimental food group that is being assessed.

Step 3: Sharing is Caring

The Whole Foods Diet has a very robust community of inspiring individuals whose lives were completely changed through a Whole Foods diet.

Once you are done tallying and recording the amazing changes that have occurred in your life, the best step to do next is to share your story with other Whole Foods Diet members who might be going through a similar situation such as yours.

You might be pleasantly surprised to see just how much of an impact your story might make in the life of someone else.

Regardless if your story is big or small, dramatic or simple! Just share it with your local Whole Foods Diet community or online.

Even if a single person reads it and says "Hey, he/she is just like me!"

Then you will feel proud that your story has touched another human being.

A good tip to make your story even more powerful is to add a picture that might show your amazing transformation.

Some pointers that you may include in your story may include:

- How you brought control over your food eating habits
- How Whole Foods Diet helped to eliminate various symptoms or conditions
- How the biomarkers such as triglycerides, blood pressure or blood sugar level improved
- How the Whole Foods Diet helped you to trim down your weight and gain back your confidence
- How Whole Foods diet helped you to be at peace with yourself
- How you were able to transfer the Whole Foods Diet habits to other aspects of your life and so on

The ideas are boundless! The only limiting factor here is your will to share your experience with the world.

Step 4: The journey afterward

You should always take the 30-day Whole Foods journey as a starting point for something great in your life. This diet won't help you completely eradicate the damage that has already been done to your body by past food decision.

However, it can surely help you rectify your mistakes and ensure that your body stays in tip-top shape in the coming days.

But let's face it, we are human beings, and at some point, we are bound to lose ourselves to the temptation of savory and delightful meals, right?

What should you do then? It is not always possible to stick to a plan like a robot!

Therefore, a good strategy moving forward should include the following steps:

- Keep focusing on your Whole Foods based meals every single day as long as you can without breaks or any "Cheat Day." Should the lust for sugar come creeping back to you, go for something very minute, just enough to control the temptation. But don't give it!
- However, should you stumble upon something that is just too irresistible or something that is culturally or religiously important to you, make a small exception and assess if the food is worth it? If it helps, then you can follow the below given that it will help you assess the food and decide if eating it would be a good idea.
- In the case where you have decided to indulge the meal, take your time to savor it. Eat consciously without ruining your diet. A good way is to eat just as much as you need to ensure that you are not feeling uncomfortable anymore and keep the rest for later use.
- Once you are done with your meal, don't feel guilt or shame! These things happen. Tell yourself that you have made a conscious decision and given yourself some slack. Moving forward, try to bring more control and stick to your Whole Foods diet as much as you can.

Word to the wise

Sometimes in your life, you might come across various occasions where eating savory food is unavoidable. Maybe during a vacation or even during a stressful time!

An easy way to get back from such sudden "Dirty" food eating sessions is to simply go on a shorter diet with a very strict Whole Foods compliant meal to get your body back on the track.

You may go on a 14-day Whole Foods or even 7-day Whole Foods diet, whichever helps you to remove the feeling of guilt and make you feel awesome again!

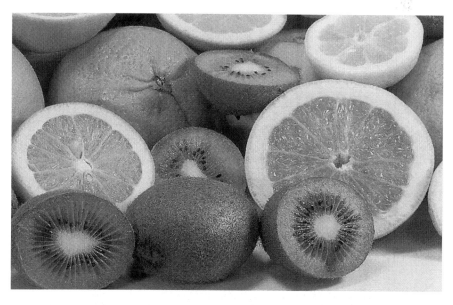

Chapter 6: Some Tips and Side Effect You Should Know About!

With all of that out of the way, here are some bonus tips for you to ensure that you can fully enjoy your Whole Foods diet as efficiently as possible!

Some tips to know about

- Always make sure to read the labels before you eat anything to ensure that you are not eating anything that is not Whole Foods Diet compliant
- Try to plan your meals for the next few days as early as possible. It will help you stay less stressed and make life easier for you
- Try to share your experience and your Whole Foods journey with as many friends and family members as you can. You may not realize it now, but a little support from loved ones will go a long way
- Don't replace junk foods with Whole Foods Diet compliant junk foods! Make sure to completely eliminate any junk food (Whole Foods Diet compliant or not)
- Make sure to go for Carbs, Healthy Fats, and Protein at every meal
- Try to avoid measuring your weight during the 30 days. Instead, focus on keeping your body healthy rather than the change in weight

Some side effects to know about

If you have already experimented or even explored through some different diets, then you are sure to know that every diet is accompanied by at least a minute number of side effects.

Naturally, this might make you wonder if the Whole Foods diet has any side effects as well.

The good news here is that the Whole Foods diet does not necessarily pose any serious threat to the body! However, there have been reports of some very minor symptoms that are experienced by newcomers.

Below, I will list them so that you may rest comfortably, knowing that they will soon pass away.

These symptoms usually show up within the first 14 days of the diet and soon go away once the body habituates itself to the new diet:

- Minor headaches
- Feeling of lethargy
- Sleepiness
- General Crankiness
- Brain Fog
- Food Cravings
- Minor Breakouts
- Minor Bloating

With all of those out of the way, here are some tips which you should keep in mind to make your Whole Foods journey as pleasant as possible.

Part 2: The Fundamentals of Vegan Diet

Throughout this part, you will find information covering topics such as:

- The basic definition of the Vegan Diet
- The variations of Vegan Diet
- The basic guidelines of the Vegan Diet
- The restrictions of the diet and the food groups you are allowed to eat and the ones you are required to get rid of.
- The side effects you should be aware of
- The advantages of following a Vegan Diet

Chapter 7: Understanding the Vegan diet

A Vegan Diet is one of the more restrictive diets out there and maintaining all of the rules might be slightly difficult in the beginning. However, that is not to say that it is impossible!

The diet altogether won't only improve your health, but will also largely decrease animal cruelty and suffering!

But before going deeper, let me first discuss what the word "Vegan" actually means.

The meaning of "Vegan"

Generally speaking, Vegan diet is a type of diet that encourages an individual to exclude any and every kind of ingredients that are animal based.

That means, aside from meat, eggs, milk and even cheese are completely off the table.

A person who follows a Vegan diet does not only follow it for the sake of staying healthy though! Veganism is nothing short of a lifestyle that encourages a revolution against animal cruelty and exploitation.

At this point, you should be aware that there is actually a considerable amount of difference between Veganism and Vegetarianism.

The people who follow a Vegan diet often tend to consider themselves as being children of nature, and they appreciate whatever Mother Nature has to offer.

As mentioned before, individuals who follow a Vegan diet tend to completely restrict themselves from having any animal/dairy products or anything that is even remotely related to animals.

On the other hand, Vegetarians allow a degree of freedom in this matter by allowing animal-derived products such as milk or eggs.

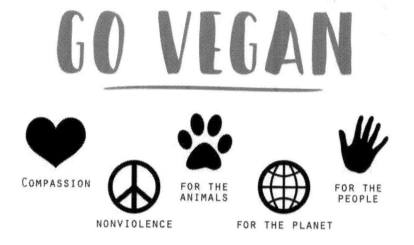

GO VEGAN

COMPASSION NONVIOLENCE FOR THE ANIMALS FOR THE PLANET FOR THE PEOPLE

The variations of Vegan Diet

Being a Vegan, you should be aware that there are actually different types of Vegan diets that are crafted by keeping the core of the intact and bringing slight variations.

These different variations of Vegan diet are designed to cater the requirement of different individuals.

While there is lot more than the ones mentioned below, these are the more famous ones

- *Whole Foods Vegan Diet:* This form of diet emphasizes on eating whole, unprocessed foods.
- *Raw-Food Vegan Diet:* This diet is primarily composed of nuts, plant foods, raw fruits, vegetable seeds that are cooked at about 118 degrees Fahrenheit.
- *80/10/10:* Also known as "Fruitarian Diet", this diet influences an individual to fully rely on fat rich plants such as avocados and nuts while relying more on raw fruits and tender greens.
- *The Starch Solution:* This is similar to the Fruitarian above diet with the exception that it focuses on cooked starches such as rice, potatoes, and corn instead of raw fruits.
- *Raw Till 4:* This low-fat diet comes as a variation from the Starch Solution diet in the sense that here you are only allowed to go for Raw Fruit up until 4 pm, after which you may go for other plant-based meals.
- *Junk Food Vegan Diet:* For those of you who just can't get away from junk foods, this is the perfect one! As this Vegan diet consists of various "Mock Meats" such as vegan cheese, fries, and desserts.

Despite the minute differences between the types, though, the main aim always remains to eliminate the meat from the diet and go for the healthy greens.

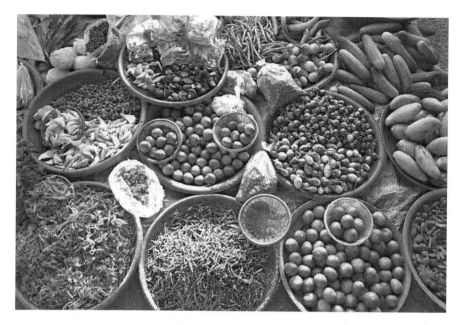

Chapter 8: The Basic Guidelines of the Vegan Diet

The basic guidelines

If you feel overwhelmed by the myriad of options provided in the previous part, you can just follow the pointers below and start your Vegan Journey.

These are the most fundamental steps that one is expected to follow if he/she is interested in following the diet.

- Make sure to eat at least five portions of vegetables and fruits that are packed with a lot of variation
- Include potatoes and other starchy carbs as your base meals to ensure that you are being provided with enough energy for the day
- Make sure to go for dairy alternatives such as yogurt, soy drink, and other low-fat alternatives
- Ensure that you are supplied with enough quantity of protein.
- If using oil and spreads, make sure to go for unsaturated ones and in small portions.
- Make sure to keep yourself packed with lots of fluid, preferably 6-8 cups per day.

When looking at the dietary routine below, you should again keep in mind that there are certain items such "Tofu" or "Legumes" that are allowed in the Vegan diet but restricted by the Whole Foods diet.

The following is yet again a generalize food list for Vegan dieticians, you are to ignore anything that goes against your Whole Foods routine.

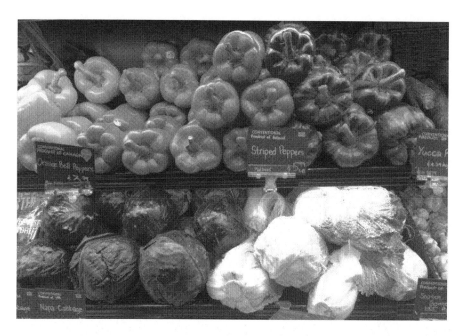

Allowed Foods

- ***Tofu, Seitan, and Tempeh:*** These are really good sources of protein and act as amazing alternatives to fish, meat, and poultry. *Warning! Not allowed in Whole Foods Diet!*
- ***Legumes:*** Legumes such as beans, peas, lentils are good sources of essential plant nutrients. *Warning! Not allowed in Whole Foods Diet!*
- ***Nuts and Nut Butters:*** Go for pure unroasted and un-blanched ones, as they are packed with selenium, zinc, fiber, iron, etc.
- ***Seeds:*** Seeds such as Flaxseed, chia, and hemp are good choices as they are packed with Omega-3 fatty acids and protein.
- ***Algae:*** Chlorella and Spirulina are good choices when it comes to seeking out good sources of protein packed Algae.

- **Calcium Fortified Plant Milks and Yogurts:** Calcium is very important to make sure that your bones are healthy! Therefore, keep the Plant-based milk and yogurts in your diet to make sure that your bones are cool. *Warning! Not allowed in Whole Foods Diet!*
- **Nutritional Yeast:** These are yet another means of easily obtaining a large amount of protein from Vegan meals. Make sure to go for the ones that are labeled "Vitamin B12" fortified for maximum benefit. *Warning! Not allowed in Whole Foods Diet!*
- **Sprouted and Fermented Plant Foods:** Tempeh, miso, natto, kombucha, and Kimchi all fall into this category, and they are packed with K2 vitamins and a good amount of probiotics. *Warning! Not allowed in Whole Foods Diet!*
- **Whole Grain Cereals and Pseudocereals:** These are good providers of complex carbs, iron, and Vitamin B. *Warning! Not allowed in Whole Foods Diet!*
- **Vegetables and Fruits:** Generally speaking, any and every vegetable and fruits are allowed on a Vegan diet! Just go wild, nature is your buffet!

Foods to avoid

- **Fish and Seafood:** All types of seafood are restricted including squid, shrimp, anchovies, calamari, crab, etc.
- **Eggs:** Any eggs, including ostrich, quail, chicken, and fish are off the table.
- **Dairy:** Ice Cream, cheese, cream, milk, and butter are restricted.
- **Animal Based Produces and Ingredients:** Such as whey, lactose, casein, egg white albumen, carmine, gelatin, etc. are to be avoided.

- *Bee Products:* Such as royal jelly, pollen, honey, etc. are to be avoided as well.
- *Meat:* Lamb, beef, horse, veal, organ meat, chicken, wild meat, goose, turkey, quail, duck, etc.

Amazing advantages of being a Vegan

- The diet will protect your body from various chronic diseases such as Type 2 Diabetes
- Help you lower down the possibility of suffering from Cardiovascular diseases or Ischemic heart diseases
- Help you relieve you from your stress and hypertension
- Protect your brain and decrease the possibility of suffering from a stroke, not to mention it will minimize the chance of you developing Alzheimer's
- The diet will help you avoid becoming obese
- You will be protected from cancers as well, including prostate and colon cancers
- A Vegan diet will keep your bones healthy and prevent arthritis
- The diet will keep your kidney in healthy condition

And those are just the beginning!

Chapter 9: Understanding the Risks of a Vegan Diet

A note on the risks of the diet

Being a Vegan will encourage you to enjoy meals that are completely based vegetables and other green goodies! However, it should be noted that the human body requires a good amount of minerals and nutrients to keep it from falling flat and stay in healthy and working order.

Naturally, the human body is habituated to an omnivorous diet so when you are going on a Vegan diet, it becomes difficult for the body to get all of the nutrients.

Therefore, it is highly recommended that you prepare a well-defined vegan plan before going on the diet. Otherwise, your body might suffer from certain vitamin and mineral deficiencies.

Since Vegan tends to replace all of the processed food with a plant-based alternative, individuals tend to grow a risk of suffering from various deficiencies such as Vitamin B12, Vitamin 2, Omega 3 and so on.

Not to worry though! There are some very specific tips and tricks that you should keep in mind while creating your diet plans to ensure that you are getting a wholly balanced Vegan meal.

And just to clear things up, Vegans are actually allowed to take supplements as well to make up for their deficiencies. Sometimes it becomes tough for an individual to properly follow all of the rules.

- *Vitamin B12:* Try to take supplements that contain B12 in cyanocobalamin form for maximum effectiveness.
- *Vitamin D:* Go for D2 or Vegan D3 that are manufactured by Viridian or Nordic Naturals.
- *EPA and DHA:* Take from algae oil.
- *Iron:* Should only be ingested using supplements should you face deficiency. Otherwise, avoid taking extra Iron.
- *Iodine:* Either take supplements or add ½ a teaspoon of iodized salt to your daily diet.
- *Calcium:* Take tablets of 500mg or less daily.

- **Zinc:** Take in forms of Zinc Citrate or Zinc Gluconate. Make sure that you are not to take these while taking Calcium supplements.

Oils to provide you with enough Fat

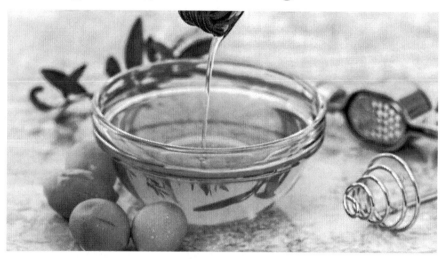

That being said, if you want to keep your fat levels in check, the following will help you.

The following oils will help you stay in line

- Coconut oil
- Olive Oil
- Avocado Oil
- Red Palm Oil
- MCT Oil
- Nuts
- Seeds
- Vegan Dairy Substitute

It should be noted that you are not allowed to have any Dairy products while on Whole Foods Diet, so you are to skip Vegan substitutes as well. Also, when it comes to nuts, make sure to avoid peanut.

Part 3: Bringing the Best of Both Worlds

While the previous 2 parts talked extensively about both of the Whole Foods diet and the Vegan diet in details, this part will give you some notes on what you should remember when trying to combine both worlds.

So, before moving forward, let me clarify one thing first.

It is not possible to fully and properly follow up on a Whole Foods diet since you will only be eating vegetables, fruits, nuts, seeds, etc. which doesn't really cover all the bases of the Whole Foods Diet.

However, that doesn't mean you won't be able to reap the benefits of the diet!

The following section will elaborate on how you will be able to slightly modify your vegan lifestyle to better incorporate the Whole Foods program within it.

First, let's start off by having a look at the benefits that you might enjoy when combining both of the diets.

Chapter 10: The advantages of a Whole Foods Vegan Diet

- Since you will be staying on a diet that is full of Anti-Oxidants and Vitamins, you will be able to enjoy the anti-inflammatory properties of the veggies and fruits.
- Since the diet will help you lower down your inflammation, it will also, in turn, support the health of your heart. The high fiber diet will protect your body from heart diseases, diabetes, cholesterol and so on.

- Since you will be eliminating junk foods, fatty food, and processed foods from your diet regime, you will be at very low risk of suffering from obesity, and it will lower down your BMI status, lowering your weight over time.
- The amount of raw foods you consume will increase drastically, and this will give you a higher number of enzymes that will help your body to break down complex food into smaller units.
- Since you are completely eliminating meat from your diet, you will be saving your body from additives and byproducts that are found in cooked and processed meats.
- The overall changes will give you a fantastic mood and minimize the feeling of lethargy and keep you active all throughout the day.
- Not to mention, the diet will help you save the environment!

And a whole lot more!

That being said, I do believe that you should have a good idea of how the combined set of rules might look like.

The combined rule set

- Sugar or any sweeteners are to be eliminated from your diet
- You are prevented from taking alcohol
- You are restricted to go for wheat, oats, rye, barley, rice, quinoa, etc. Simply put, grains are off the table
- No legumes such as beans, peanuts, lentils are allowed
- Dairy products are not allowed
- And of course, meats are off the table due to the Vegan way of the life

Protein Source

When you start and include Vegan diet in your life, most of the people could have misconceptions concerning protein deficiency because protein will play an essential role to build and maintain tissues. But we can get the right amount of protein for our body by consuming plant-based food products also.

If you feel that you require additional protein for your body, feel free to add plant-based protein powder in your food or juices or smoothies (some of the plant-based protein powder are pea protein powder, hemp protein powder, pumpkin protein powder, cranberry protein powder, and so on).

Chapter 11: How to adjust the Whole Foods Diet for Vegans

Before going into the Whole Foods Vegan diet, you should keep your expectations in check first!

Following a Whole Foods Vegan Diet, you won't be able to completely reset your body to the fullest. However, you will be able to bring your health to a significantly better condition.

The inclusion of the various plant-based protein sources is known to have some negative impacts on hormonal balance, immune system, digestive tracts, etc. due to the lack of certain nutrients and proteins, which the body would've gotten through an animal-based diet.

However, it is possible to tackle these and by following a well-balanced diet and take supplements if necessary (already discussed in the Vegan Diet part).

That being said, let me elaborate on how you can modify the general Whole Foods diet to better suit your needs.

Firstly, you should keep in mind that the idea of "Protein-Combining" is way out of date and you should appreciate the fact that your body has the capacity to store amino acids from the food you eat for a day or two.

So, make sure to eat a wide variety of plant-based proteins to keep things fresh and interesting.

Good choices include fermented soy products such as tempeh, natto, organic Edamame, organic soy like tofu and so on.

Many kinds of hemp/pea protein powder are also good options as well when you might feel like your protein levels are low.

Now you may have already noticed that the rules mentioned above go directly against the typical Whole Foods diet, which might seem a bit crazy at first!

But this was the rule set to welcome the Vegan community with open arms.

It is impossible to follow the Whole Foods diet without protein. And soy, some legumes, etc. are the best way to get protein while on a Vegan diet, therefore the cuts were made on this front.

However, you are still highly encouraged to avoid any kind of grain!

With all of that out of the way, you should know that the recipes provided in this book follow a more traditional route and try to combine the traditional vegan and Whole Foods diets as much as possible

with little to no deviation (unless absolutely necessary).

So, feel free to explore the recipes and adjust them according to your desired regime!

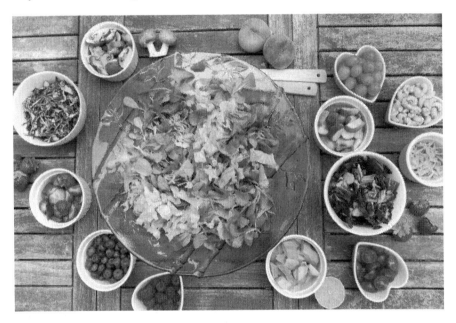

Part 4: Finally, the Recipes!

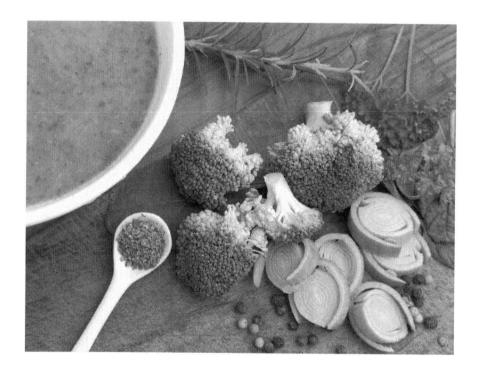

Chapter 12: Breakfast Recipes

Roasted Cauliflower Soup

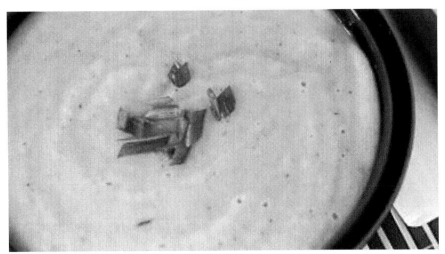

Serves: 6

Prep Time: 15 minutes

Cook Time: 60 minutes

Ingredients

- 2 cauliflower head broken up into florets
- Olive oil cooking spray
- ¼ cup of olive oil
- 1 chopped up a large onion
- 4 cloves of chopped up garlic
- 6 cups of water
- Salt as needed
- Pepper as needed

Directions

1. Add cauliflower florets to a large-sized bowl filled with salty water
2. Allow it to sit for 20 minutes
3. Drain and arrange them on a sheet of aluminum foil on your baking sheet
4. Spray olive oil evenly over the cauliflower
5. Pre-heat your broiler to high and set the rack 6 inch away from the heat source
6. Broil for 20-30 minutes
7. Take a large soup pot and place it over medium heat
8. Add onion and cook for 5 minutes
9. Stir in garlic, roasted cauliflower and water and cook for 30 minutes
10. Blend the soup using an immersion blender and serve!

Nutritional Values per Serving

- Calories: 140
- Fat: 10g
- Carbohydrates: 13g
- Protein: 4g

All-Star Baked Apple

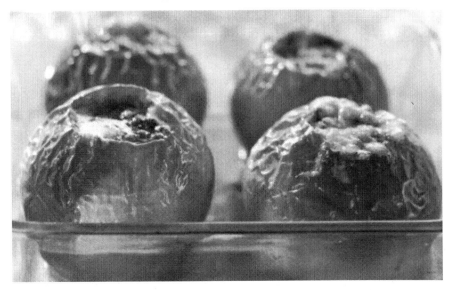

Serves: 1

Prep Time: 5 minutes

Cook Time: 20 minutes

Ingredients

- 4 pieces of Fuji apple
- Raisins as needed
- Cinnamon as needed

Directions

1. Pre-heat your oven to 347 degrees Fahrenheit
2. Core the apples
3. Stuff them with cinnamon and raisins
4. Transfer to the oven and bake for 20 minutes
5. Serve and enjoy!

Nutritional Values per Serving

- Calories: 95
- Fat: 0.27g
- Carbohydrates: 42g
- Protein: 0.43g

Banana Bites

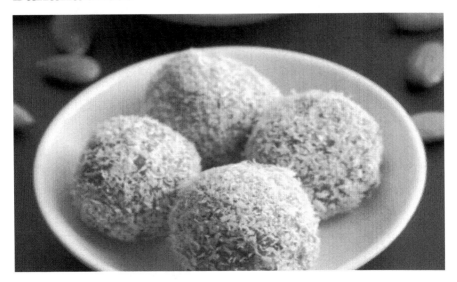

Serves: 4

Prep Time: 10 minutes

Cook Time: 0 minute

Ingredients

- 4 teaspoon of cocoa powder (unsweetened)
- 4 teaspoon of toasted unsweetened coconut
- 2 sliced of small bananas

Directions

1. Take two individual plates and place the cocoa and coconut on those plates (individually)
2. Roll up the banana slices in the cocoa first and shake off any excess
3. Then dip them in the coconut
4. Serve!

Nutrition Values (per Serving)

- Protein: 1g
- Carbs: 13g
- Fats: 1g
- Calories: 60

Healthy Banana Smoothie

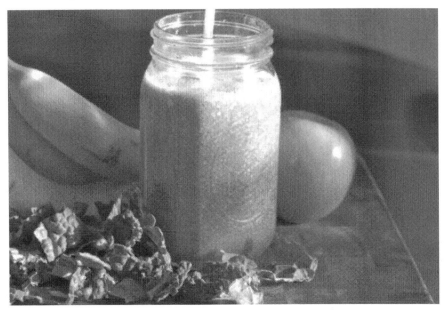

Serves: 1

Prep Time: 5 minutes

Cook Time: 0 minutes

Ingredients

- 1 piece of banana
- 2 cups of chopped kale
- ½ a cup of light unsweetened almond milk
- 1 tablespoon of flax seed

Directions

1. Add the listed ingredients to your blender and blend them
2. Once you have a smooth mixture, chill and serve!

Nutritional Values per Serving

- Calories: 311
- Fat: 7.3g
- Carbohydrates: 56g
- Protein: 12g

Easy Carrot Balls

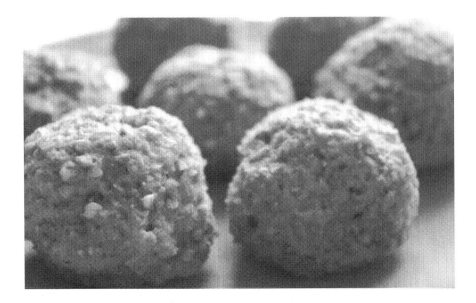

Serves: 10

Prep Time: 10 minutes

Cook Time: 0 minutes

Ingredients

- 6 pieces of pitted Medjool dates
- 1 finely grated carrot
- ¼ cup of raw walnuts
- ¼ cup of unsweetened finely shredded coconut
- 1 teaspoon of nutmeg
- 1/8 teaspoon of sea salt

Directions

1. Take a food processor and add dates, ¼ cup of grated carrots, salt coconut, nutmeg
2. Mix well and puree the mixture

3. Add the walnuts and remaining ¼ cup of carrots
4. Pulse the mixture until you have a chunky texture
5. Form balls using your hand and roll them up in coconut
6. Top with carrots and chill
7. Enjoy!

Nutritional Values per Serving

- Calories: 326
- Fat: 16g
- Carbohydrates: 42g
- Protein: 3g

Goodmorning Avocado Spread

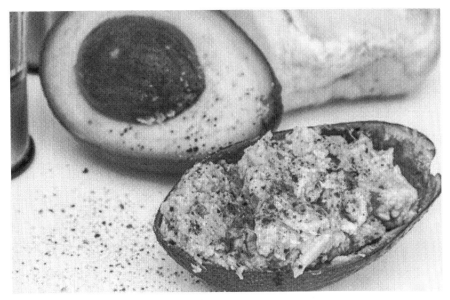

Serves: 4

Prep Time: 10 minutes

Cook Time: 0 minutes

Ingredients

- 1 halved and pitted avocado
- 2 tablespoon of chopped fresh parsley
- 1 and a ½ teaspoon of extra virgin olive oil
- ½ a lemon juice
- ½ a teaspoon of salt
- ½ a teaspoon of ground black pepper
- ½ a teaspoon of onion powder
- ½ a teaspoon of garlic powder

Directions

1. Scoop out the avocado flesh into a bowl

2. Add lemon juice, parsley, olive oil, salt, onion powder, garlic, and pepper
3. Mix well and mash the mixture using potato masher
4. Serve the avocado spread as you like
5. Enjoy!

Nutritional Values per Serving

- Calories: 170
- Fat: 10g
- Carbohydrates: 16g
- Protein: 5g

Almond Berry Smoothie

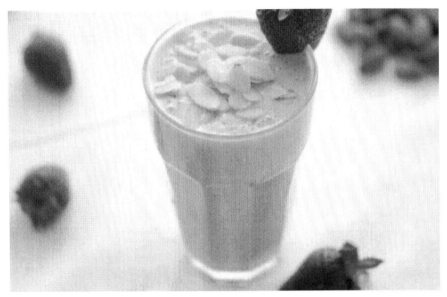

Serves: 4

Prep Time: 10 minutes

Cook Time: 0 minutes

Ingredients

- 1 cup of frozen blueberries
- 1 piece of banana
- ½ a cup of almond milk
- 1 tablespoon of almond butter (Whole Foods Compliant Brand)
- Water as needed

Directions

1. Add the listed ingredients to the blender and blend them well until you have a smooth texture
2. Add water to thin out the smoothie

3. Chill and enjoy!

Nutritional Values per Serving

- Calories: 321
- Fat: 11g
- Carbohydrates: 55g
- Protein: 5.3g

Easy Coconut Date Bars

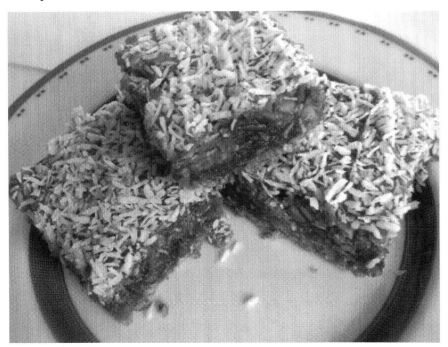

<u>**Serves:**</u> **4**

<u>**Prep Time:**</u> **10 minutes**

<u>**Cook Time:**</u> **30 minutes**

- 1/3 cup of slivered almonds
- ½ a cup of flaked coconut
- 10 pieces of pitted dates
- ¼ cup of cashews
- 1 teaspoon of coconut oil

<u>Directions</u>

1. Add almonds to your food processor and blend them
2. Add dates and pulse until well mixed
3. Add coconut oil, cashew and mix until you have a thick mixture

4. Transfer the mix to wax paper and form squares
5. Fold the squares and chill for 30 minutes
6. Serve!

<u>Nutritional Values per Serving</u>

- Calories: 154
- Fats: 0g
- Carbs: 39g
- Protein: 0.1g

Delicious Cucumber and Pear Smoothie

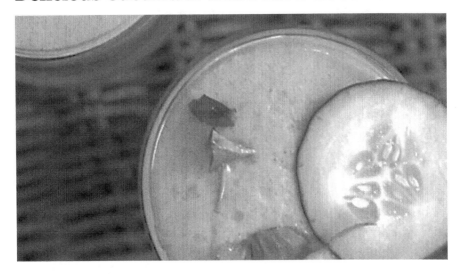

Serves: 2

Prep Time: 10 minutes

Cook Time: 0 minutes

Ingredients

- ¼ cup chopped up cucumber
- 1 chopped up pear
- ¼ cup of frozen pineapple
- 1 tablespoon of chopped up fresh parsley
- ½ a teaspoon of grated fresh ginger
- ½ a cup of water

Directions

1. Layer your cucumber, pineapple, parsley, white beans, ginger, pears in your blender
2. Add water and cover
3. Blend until you have a smooth mixture
4. Serve and enjoy!

Nutritional Values per Serving

- Calories: 167
- Fat: 0.5g
- Carbohydrates: 41g
- Protein: 3.8g

Salty Almond Butter Bites

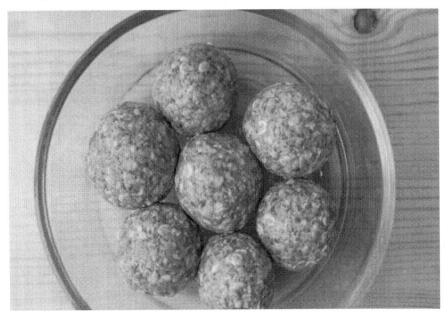

Serves: 9

Prep Time: 15 minutes

Cook Time: 0 minutes

Ingredients

- 1 cup of raw almonds
- ½ a cup of Almond butter
- 1 cup of pitted Medjool dates
- 1 and a ¼ teaspoon of vanilla bean extract
- Sea salt as needed

Directions

1. Take a food processor and add almonds, almond butter, vanilla, dates and blend the whole mixture until a dough-like texture comes (should take a few minutes)
2. Add some more almond butter if you want a stickier dough

3. Form balls using the dough and press down using fork to create a criss-cross pattern
4. Sprinkle salt generously
5. Serve immediately or allow it to chill for crunchiness

Nutritional Values per Serving

- Calories: 350
- Fat: 17g
- Carbohydrates: 27g
- Protein: 18g

Fried Apples

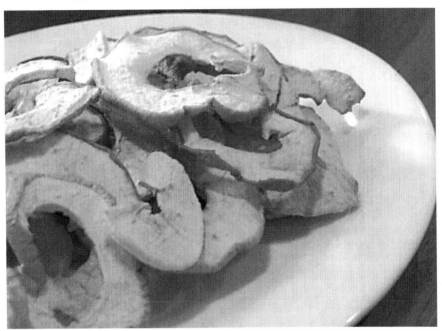

Serves: 4

Prep Time: 10 minutes

Cook Time: 10 minute

Ingredients

- ½ a cup of coconut oil
- ¼ cup of date paste
- 2 tablespoon of ground cinnamon
- 4 pieces of Granny Smith Apples, peeled, sliced and cored

Directions

1. Take a large sized skillet and place it over medium heat
2. Add oil and allow it to heat up
3. Stir in cinnamon and date paste into the oil

4. Add the cut up apples and cook them nicely for about 5-8 minutes until they break down
5. Enjoy!

Nutritional Values per Serving

- Calories: 369
- Fat: 23g
- Carbohydrates: 44g
- Protein: 1g

Plums From the Oven

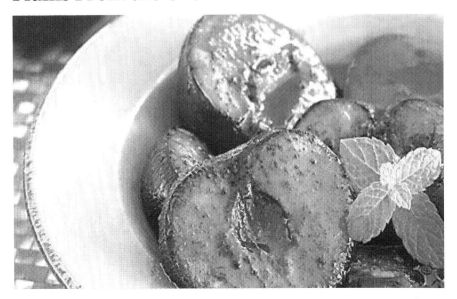

Serves: 3

Prep Time: 10 minutes

Cook Time: 15 minutes

- 4 pieces of plums, pitted and halved
- ½ a cup of orange juice
- 2 tablespoon of date paste
- ½ a teaspoon of ground cinnamon
- 1/8 teaspoon of ground nutmeg
- 1/8 teaspoon of cumin
- 1/8 teaspoon of cardamom
- ¼ cup of toasted and slivered almonds

Directions

1. Pre-heat your oven to 400 degrees Fahrenheit
2. Take a shallow baking dish and grease it with cooking spray
3. Add plums to the pan with the cut side facing up

4. Take a bowl and whisk in orange juice, date paste, cinnamon, cumin, cardamom, and nutmeg
5. Drizzle the mix over the plums
6. Bake for 20 minutes and top it up with some slivered almonds
7. Serve!

Nutritional Values per Serving

- Calories: 113
- Fats: 4g
- Carbs: 20g
- Protein: 2.1g

Eggplant and Tomato Soup

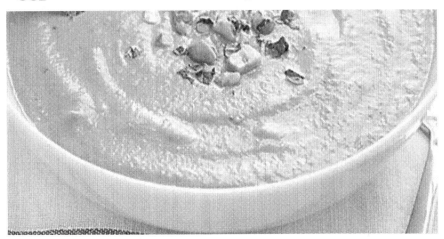

Serves: 6

Prep Time: 10 minutes

Cook Time: 25 minutes

- 1 medium-sized eggplant dice up 1-inch cubes
- 5 large sized cored and diced tomatoes
- 1 cup roughly chopped up yellow onion
- 3 garlic cloves
- ¼ cup of extra virgin olive oil
- Salt as needed
- Pepper as needed
- ½ a cup of raw cashews soaked overnight
- 1 and a ½ cup of vegetable broth
- 1 tablespoon fresh oregano
- 1 tablespoon of fresh basil

Directions

1. Pre-heat your oven to 400 degrees Fahrenheit
2. Take two baking sheets and line them up with parchment paper

3. Divide the eggplant, onion, tomatoes, garlic amongst the baking sheets

4. Pour half of your olive oil onto each and sprinkle pepper and salt

5. Take a spoon and stir the veggies until they are coated with oil

6. Transfer to the baking sheet into your pre-heated oven and bake for 20 minutes

7. Remove and allow them to cool

8. Once the veggies are cool, transfer them to your blender

9. Drain the cashews and add them to the blender as well

10. Add vegetable broth, herbs and blend on high speed

11. Reheat in your microwave and serve with a garnish of chopped up cashews

12. Enjoy!

<u>Nutritional Values per Serving</u>

- Calories: 266
- Fats: 4g
- Carbs: 47g
- Protein: 10g

Avocado and Banana Smoothie

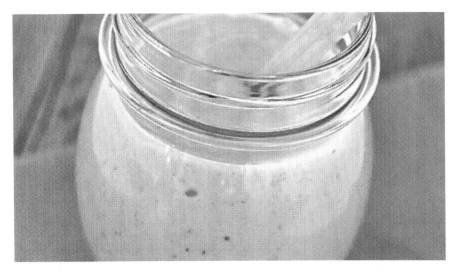

Serves: 1

Prep Time: 10 minutes

Cook Time: 0 minutes

Ingredients

- 1 cup of almond milk
- 1 peeled and pitted avocado
- 1 large sized banana cut up into chunks
- 3 tablespoon of creamy cashew butter
- 2 ice cubes

Directions

1. Add all of the ingredients to a blender and blend well until you have a nice and smooth texture
2. Serve chilled!

Nutritional Values per Serving

- Calories: 806

- Fat: 57g
- Carbohydrates: 66g
- Protein: 18g

Match Dredged Coconut Smoothie

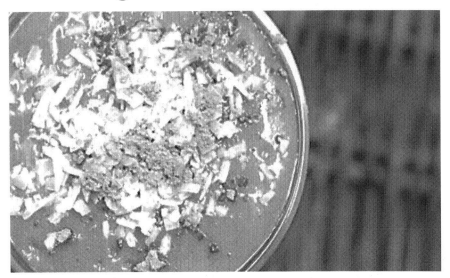

Serves: 2

Prep Time: 10 minutes

Cook Time: 0 minutes

Ingredients

- 1 piece of banana
- 1 cup of frozen mango chunks
- 2 kale leaves torn up into several pieces
- 2 tablespoon of shredded coconut
- ½ a teaspoon of matcha green tea powder
- 1 cup of water

Directions

1. Add banana, kale, mango, matcha powder and white beans to the blender
2. Blend until you have a nice smoothie
3. Serve and enjoy!

Nutritional Values per Serving

- Calories: 367
- Fat: 8g
- Carbohydrates: 72g
- Protein: 8g

Pumpkin Butter Nut Cup

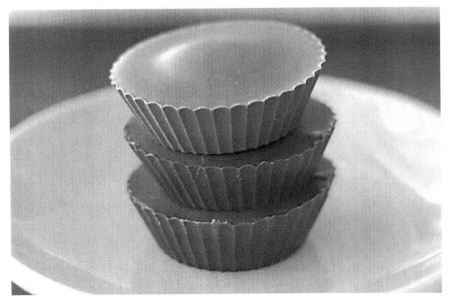

<u>Serves:</u> 5

<u>Prep Time:</u> 135 minutes

<u>Cook Time:</u> 0 minute

For Filing

- ½ a cup of organic pumpkin puree
- 1/2a cup of homemade almond butter
- 4 tablespoon of organic coconut oil
- ¼ teaspoon of organic ground nutmeg
- ¼ teaspoon of organic ground ginger
- 1 teaspoon of organic ground cinnamon
- 1/8 teaspoon of organic ground clove
- 2 teaspoon of organic vanilla bean extract

For Topping

- 1 cup of organic raw cacao powder

- 1 cup of organic coconut oil

Directions

1. Take a medium-sized bowl and add all of the listed ingredients under pumpkin filling
2. Mix well until you have a creamy mixture
3. Take another bowl and add the topping mixture and mix well
4. Take a muffin cup and fill it up with 1/3 of the chocolate topping mix
5. Chill for 15 minutes
6. Add 1/3 of the pumpkin mix and layer out on top
7. Chill for 2 hours
8. Repeat until all the mixture has been used up
9. Enjoy!

Nutritional Values per Serving

- Calories: 105
- Fat: 10.1g
- Carbohydrates: 3.3g
- Protein: 2.9g

Green Smoothie

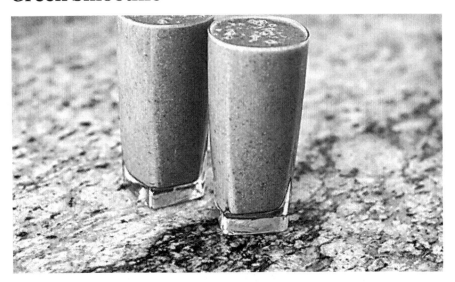

Serves: 1

Prep Time: 10 minutes

Cook Time: 0 minute

- 1 cup of frozen mixed berries
- ½ a cup of baby spinach leaves
- 2 tablespoon of fresh orange juice
- 2 tablespoon of water
- 1 medium-sized ripe banana sliced up

Directions

1. Open up the lid of your food processor
2. Add all of the listed ingredients into the blender/food processor
3. Blend everything well until a smooth consistency comes
4. Serve chilled!

Nutritional Values per Serving

- Protein: 18g

- Carbs: 54g
- Fats: 3.8g
- Calories: 297

Sunny Smoothie

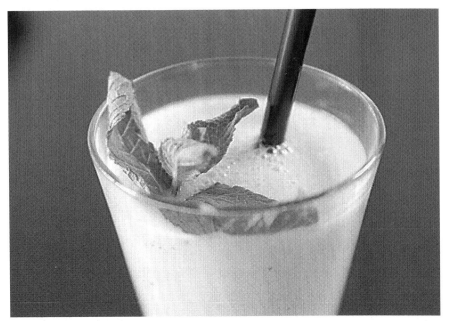

Prep Time: 5 minutes

Cooking Time: 30 minute

Serves: 4

Ingredients:

- ½ of a frozen banana
- ½ a cup of fresh orange juice
- ¾ cup of frozen mango
- ¼ cup of water

Portion 2

- ½ of a frozen banana
- ¾ cup of frozen strawberries
- ½ a cup of water
- a few ice cubes

Directions:

1. Notice that here the ingredients here are divided into two portions. Firstly blend up all of the ingredients listed in portion one and set it aside
2. Then take all of the ingredients of portion 2 and blend them up.
3. Pour half of the portion 2 mixture into the cup of portion 1 and mix them together
4. Once an orange-pinkish texture has been achieved, very slowly pour the mixture into the cup with portion 1
5. Then take the portion 2 mixture and set it aside only to slowly pour it into a cup
6. And you are done!

Nutritional Values per Serving

- Calories: 240
- Fat: 8g
- Carbohydrates: 22g
- Protein: 20g

Carrot and Banana Filled Smoothie

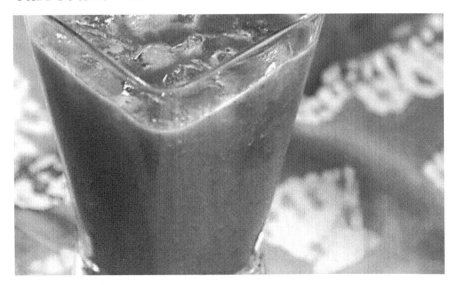

Serves: 2

Prep Time: 15 minutes

Cook Time: 0 minutes

Ingredients

- 1 piece of banana
- 1 cup chopped up cucumbers
- 2/3 cup chopped up red bell pepper
- ½ a cup of ruby-red grapefruit juice
- ½ a cup of chopped up carrots
- Ice cubes as needed

Directions

4. Add all of the listed ingredients to the blend and blend it
5. Pour the smoothie into a glass filled with ice and serve!

Nutritional Values per Serving

- Calories: 115
- Fat: 0.6g
- Carbohydrates: 27g
- Protein: 2.2g

Chapter 13: Lunch Recipes

Crispy Potatoes and Vegan Sauce

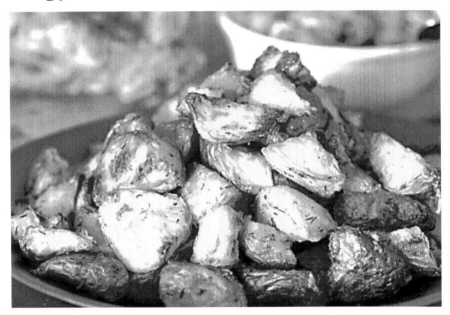

Serves: 4

Prep Time: 15 minutes

Cook Time: 30 minutes

Ingredients

- 2 pound of mixed and halved baby potatoes
- 3 tablespoon of canola oil
- 1 cup of raw unsalted cashews soaked overnight
- 3 tablespoon of lemon juice
- ½ a teaspoon of chili powder
- ½ a teaspoon of sweet paprika
- ½ a teaspoon of garlic powder
- 1 teaspoon of Coarse sea salt

- ¼ cup of nutritional yeast
- ½ of a jalapeno chili, chopped and seeded

Directions

1. Pre-heat your oven to 450 degrees Fahrenheit
2. Take a bowl and add potatoes, ½ a teaspoon of salt, ¼ teaspoon of pepper, oil
3. Take a rimmed baking sheet and spread the potatoes evenly
4. Roast for 30 minutes
5. Take a blender and add lemon juice, chili powder, cashews, paprika, cumin, garlic powder, yeast, sea salt and jalapeno
6. Add 1 cup of water
7. Puree the mix well
8. Transfer to a 2-quart saucepan and simmer for 5 minutes over low heat
9. Transfer the vegan sauce to a bowl and serve with your roast potatoes

Nutritional Values per Serving

- Calories: 380
- Fat: 18g
- Carbohydrates: 47g
- Protein: 10

Mushroom, Beet and Avocado Salad

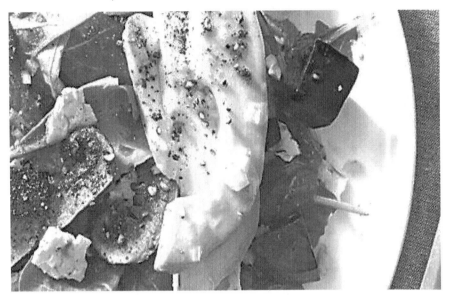

Serves: 4

Prep Time: 10 minutes

Cook Time: 20 minutes

Ingredients

- 4 medium-sized Portobello mushroom caps
- ¼ cup of lemon juice
- 3 tablespoon of olive oil
- 1 small shallots finely chopped up
- 5 ounce of baby kale
- 8 ounce of precooked, chopped up beets
- 2 thinly sliced ripe avocados

Directions

1. Take a large sized rimmed baking sheet

2. Spray the Portobello mushroom caps with cooking spray and sprinkle ½ a teaspoon of salt
3. Add mushroom to the baking sheet and bake for 20 minutes at 450 degrees Fahrenheit
4. Take a bowl and whisk in lemon juice, olive oil, shallot, ¼ teaspoon of salt, ¼ teaspoon of pepper
5. Add half of the beets and baby kale and give everything a nice toss
6. Divide the mixture amongst serving plates and top them with avocados, mushrooms
7. Serve with dressing and enjoy!

Nutritional Values per Serving

- Calories: 370
- Fat: 26g
- Carbohydrates: 32g
- Protein: 7g

Another Green Smoothie

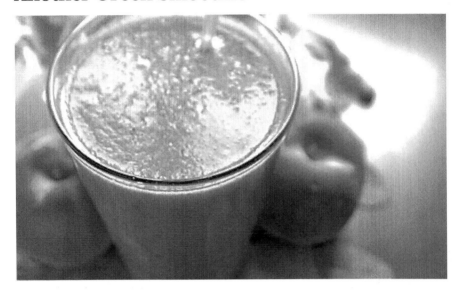

Serves: 2

Prep Time: 10 minutes

Cook Time: 0 minutes

Ingredients

- 2 cups of coconut water
- 3.5 ounce of spinach
- 1 tablespoon of almond butter
- 2 small sized bananas
- 1 teaspoon of vanilla essence
- 1 tablespoon of hemp seeds
- 1 tablespoon of chia seeds

Directions

1. Carefully place all of the ingredients into a blender and blend them well
2. Chill and serve!

Nutritional Values per Serving

- Calories: 289
- Fat: 6g
- Carbohydrates: 58g
- Protein: 6g

Grilled Guacamole Avocado

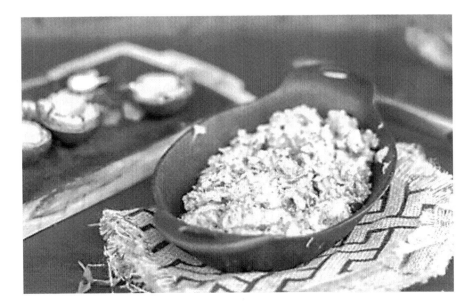

Serves: 4

Prep Time: 15 minutes

Cook Time: 5 minutes

Ingredients

- 5 whole pieces of avocados
- ¼ cup of diced red onion
- 1 whole jalapeno
- 2 cloves of garlic
- ¼ teaspoon of cumin
- ½ a teaspoon of smoked paprika
- ¼ teaspoon of salt
- ¼ teaspoon of black pepper
- ½ of a whole lime

Directions

1. Halve the avocados and place them on your grill over HIGH HEAT
2. Grill for 5 minutes until slightly charred
3. Scoop out the flesh into bowls
4. Add onion, chopped jalapeno, cumin, garlic, salt, pepper, and paprika
5. Mix well
6. Squeeze a bit of lemon juice and serve!

Nutritional Values per Serving

- Calories: 350
- Fat: 21g
- Carbohydrates: 36g
- Protein: 7g

Fancy Melon and Watercress Salad

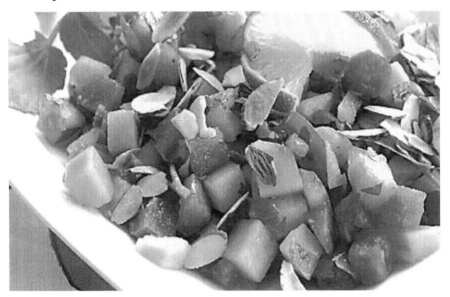

Serves: 4

Prep Time: 15 minutes

Cook Time: 0 minutes

- 3 tablespoon of fresh lime juice
- 1 teaspoon of date paste
- 1 teaspoon of minced fresh ginger root
- ¼ cup of vegetable oil
- 2 bunch of chopped up and trimmed watercress
- 2 and a ½ cups of cubed watermelon
- 2 and a ½ cups of cubed cantaloupe
- 1/3 cup of toasted and sliced almonds

Directions

1. Take a large sized bowl and add lime juice and ginger, date paste

2. Whisk well and add the oil

3. Season with salt and pepper

4. Add cantaloupe, watercress, watermelon
5. Toss and coat everything up
6. Transfer to serving bowls and garnish with sliced almonds
7. Enjoy!

Nutritional Values per Serving

- Calories: 274
- Fats: 20g
- Carbs: 21g
- Protein: 7g

Onion and Orange "Magnifique" Salad

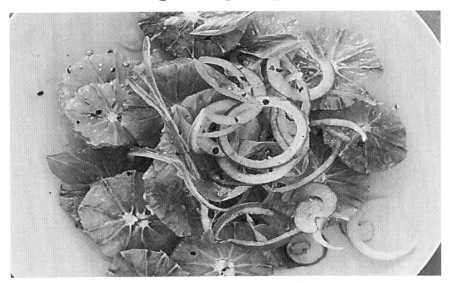

Serves: 2

Prep Time: 15 minutes

Cook Time: 15 minutes

- 6 large pieces of oranges
- 3 tablespoon of red wine vinegar
- 6 tablespoon of olive oil
- 1 teaspoon of dried oregano
- 1 red onion thinly sliced up
- 1 cup of black olives
- ¼ cup of chopped fresh chives
- Ground black pepper

Directions

1. Peel the orange and cut each of them into 4-5 crosswise slices

2. Transfer to a shallow serving dish and sprinkle vinegar, oregano, and olive oil

3. Toss well

4. Chill for 30 minutes

5. Arrange the sliced up onion and black olives on top

6. Decorate well and sprinkle some chives on top with a grind of fresh pepper

7. Enjoy!

<u>Nutritional Values per Serving</u>

- Calories: 120
- Fat: 6g
- Carbohydrates: 20g
- Protein: 2g

Frozen Salad Bowl

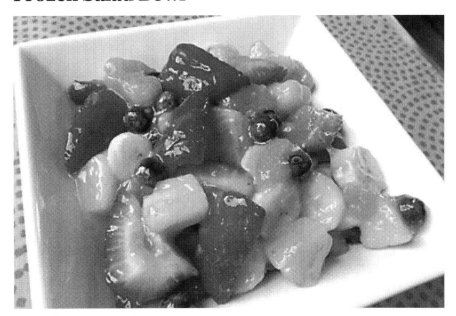

Serves: 3

Prep Time: 75 minutes

Cook Time: 0 minutes

- 2 cups of water
- ¼ cup of date paste
- 1 can of 20-ounces frozen orange juice concentrate (thawed)
- 1 can of 20-ounces frozen lemonade concentrate (thawed)
- 4 sliced up bananas
- 1 can of crushed pineapple (with juice)
- 1 pack of strawberries (thawed)

Directions

1. Take a bowl and add date paste and water

2. Mix well and add orange juice, lemonade, banana, crushed pineapple, strawberries

3. Give it a nice mix

4. Pour the mixture into 9x13 inch glass pan and chill

5. Let it sit for 5 minutes at room temp

6. Cut it out and serve!

Nutritional Values per Serving

- Calories: 350
- Fats: 0.5g
- Carbs: 89g
- Protein: 2.5g

Extremely Fresh Pineapple Salsa

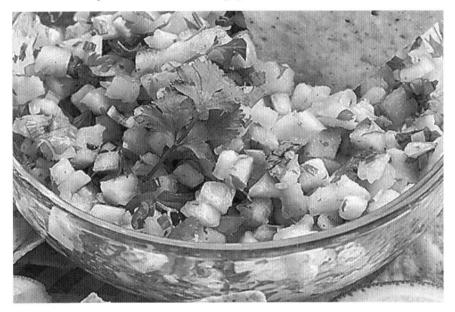

Serves: 3

Prep Time: 75 minutes

Cook Time: 0 minutes

- ½ of pineapple cut up into small diced
- 2 teaspoon of chopped fine jalapeno
- 2 thinly sliced green onion
- 1 teaspoon of ground cumin
- 2 tablespoon of freshly squeezed lime juice
- ¼ cup of cilantro chopped up
- Salt as needed
- Pepper as needed

Directions

1. Cut up the outer skin of your Pineapple by cutting off the ends
2. Stand it on one side and cut the sides flat

3. Slice the pineapple into ¼ inch planks down the side

4. Cut the planks into dices and add them to a bowl

5. Chop up the jalapeno and cut off the stem

6. Slice them lengthwise and take out the membrane and seeds and add them to the bowl

7. Slice the green onion into very thin layers and add them to the bowl

8. Add cumin, lime juice, cilantro, salt and pepper and toss well

9. Serve and enjoy!

<u>Nutritional Values per Serving</u>

- Calories: 255
- Fats: 1g
- Carbs: 64g
- Protein: 3g

Stinky Roasted Garlic

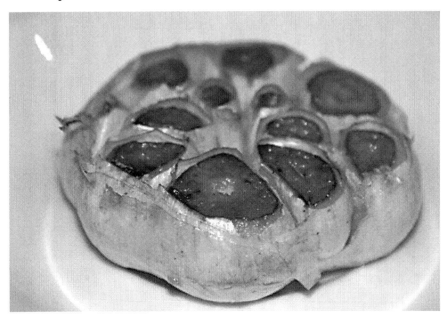

Serves: 4

Prep Time: 5 minutes

Cook Time: 20 minutes

Ingredients

- 1 medium garlic head
- 2 tablespoon of olive oil

Directions

1. Pre-heat your oven to a temperature of 250 degrees Fahrenheit
2. Peel each of your garlic clove
3. Place the cloves in a single layer in a small sized baking dish and drizzle some olive oil
4. Bake for about 15 minutes until the garlic are tender

Nutritional Values per Serving

- Calories: 81
- Fat: 7g
- Carbohydrates: 5g
- Protein: 1g

Salty Cashew Larabars

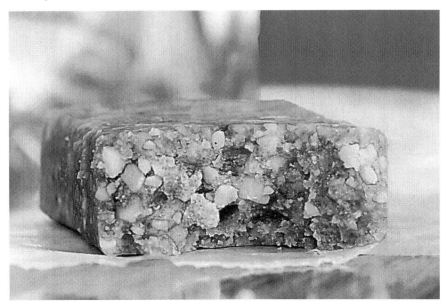

Serves: 10

Prep Time: 10 minutes

Cook Time: 10 minutes

Ingredients

- 30 finely pitted Medjool dates
- 1 and a ½ cups of raw cashews
- Just a pinch of salt

Directions

1. Take a food processor and add the dates
2. Process them until you have a nice paste
3. Add cashews and pulse until you have a coarse chopped texture and the dates have been fully mixed with the cashews
4. Use the dough to form a nice ball or square and cut it up into bars
5. Enjoy!

<u>Nutritional Values per Serving</u>

- Calories: 223
- Fat: 2g
- Carbohydrates: 55g
- Protein: 2g

Ginger and Vegetable Stir Fry

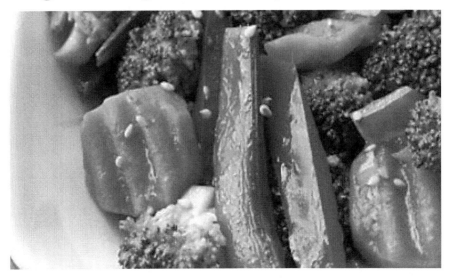

Prep Time: 25 minutes

Cooking Time: 15 minute

Serves: 7

Ingredients

- 1 tablespoon of arrowroot
- 1 and a ½ crushed cloves
- 2 teaspoon of chopped fresh ginger root
- ¼ cup of olive oil
- 1 small head of broccoli cut up into florets
- ¾ cup of julienned carrots
- ½ a cup of green beans
- 2 tablespoon of soy sauce
- 2 and a ½ tablespoon of water
- ¼ cup chopped onion
- ½ a tablespoon of salt

Directions

1. Take a large sized bowl and add arrowroot powder, 1 teaspoon of ginger, two tablespoons of olive oil and mix until the arrowroot has dissolved

2. Add broccoli, carrots, beans and toss well

3. Take a large skillet and heat up 2 tablespoons of olive oil

4. Cook the veggies for 2 minutes

5. Stir well

6. Stir in soy sauce and water

7. Add onion, salt and 1 teaspoon of ginger

8. Cook until crisp

9. Serve!

Nutritional Values per Serving

- Calories: 119
- Fat: 9g
- Carbohydrates: 8g
- Protein: 2g

Mushroom and Pepper Kabob

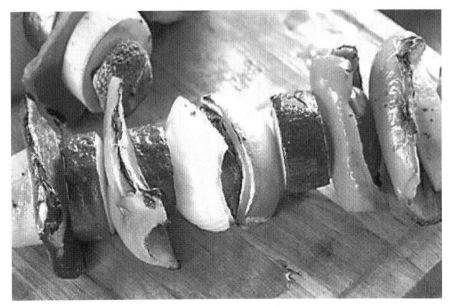

Prep Time: 30 minutes

Cooking Time: 10 minute

Serves: 4

Ingredients

- ¾ cup of sliced fresh mushrooms
- 2 red bell peppers chopped up
- 1 green bell pepper cut up into 1-inch pieces
- ¼ cup of olive oil
- 2 tablespoon of lemon juice
- 1 minced garlic clove
- 2 teaspoon of chopped fresh thyme
- 1 teaspoon of chopped fresh rosemary
- ¼ teaspoon of salt
- ¼ teaspoon of ground black pepper

Directions

1. Pre-heat your grill to medium heat
2. Thread the mushroom and pepper alternately onto skewers
3. Take a small bowl and add olive oil, lemon juice, thyme, salt, pepper, rosemary and garlic
4. Brush the mushroom and pepper with the mixture
5. Brush the grate with oil
6. Place your kabobs on grill and cook for 4-6 minutes while basting them
7. Enjoy!

Nutritional Values per Serving

- Calories: 151
- Fat: 13g
- Carbohydrates: 6.5g
- Protein: 1.4g

Zucchini "Pizza" Boats

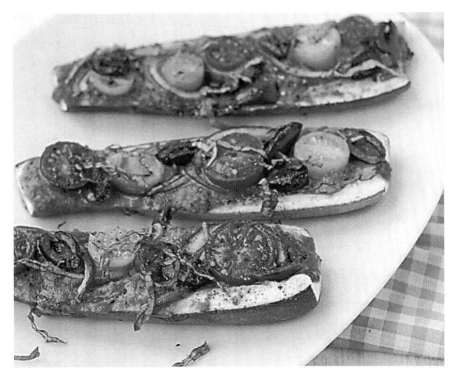

Prep Time: 10 minutes

Cooking Time: 25 minute

Serves: 4

Ingredients

- 4 pieces of medium zucchini
- ½ a cup of <u>Whole Foods</u> compliant Marinara sauce/tomato sauce
- 1/4 sliced red onion
- ¼ cup chopped kalamata olives
- ½ a cup of sliced cherry tomatoes
- 2 tablespoon of fresh basil

Directions

1. Pre-heat your oven to 400 degrees Fahrenheit
2. Cut up the Zucchini half-lengthwise and shape them in boats
3. Take a bowl and add tomato sauce
4. Spread 1 layer of the sauce on top of each boat and top with onion, tomato, and olives
5. Bake for 20-25 minutes until the Zucchini are tender
6. Top with basil and serve!

Nutritional Values per Serving

- Calories: 278
- Fat: 20g
- Carbohydrates: 10g
- Protein: 15g

Apple and Kale Soup

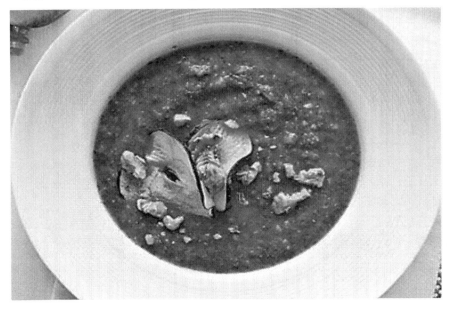

<u>**Prep Time:**</u> **20 minutes**

<u>**Cooking Time:**</u> **1 minute**

<u>**Serves:**</u> **2**

<u>**Ingredients**</u>

- 8 walnut halves broken up into pieces
- 1 finely chopped up onion
- 2 coarsely grated carrots
- 2 unpeeled but finely chopped up red apples
- 1 tablespoon of cider vinegar
- 2 cups of reduced salt vegetable stock
- 7 ounce of roughly chopped kale
- 1 ounce of dried apple crisps

Directions

1. Take a non-stick frying pan and add your walnuts, cook them for about 2-3 minutes until they are nice and toasty
2. Remove the heat and let them cool
3. Take a large sized saucepan and add carrots onion, vinegar, apples and bring the whole mixture to a boil
4. Lower down the heat and let it simmer for about 10 minutes, making sure to keep stirring it from time to time
5. Once the onion is translucent and the apples are tender, add your kale to the mixture and let it simmer for yet another 2 minutes
6. Gently transfer the whole mixture to a blender and let it blend until very smooth
7. Pour the soup into your serving bowls and garnish with some apple crisps and toasted walnuts
8. Serve!

Nutritional Values per Serving

- Protein: 12g
- Carbs: 36g
- Fats: 21g
- Calories: 403

Fresh Avocado and Cilantro Salad

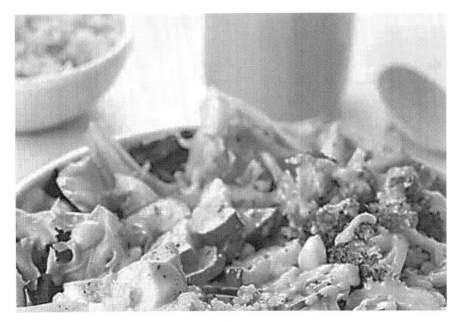

Prep Time: 10 minutes

Cooking Time: 0 minute

Serves: 6

Ingredients:

- 2 avocados – peeled, pitted and diced
- 1 chopped up sweet onion
- 1 green bell pepper (chopped up)
- 1 large sized chopped up a ripe tomato
- ¼ cup of chopped up fresh cilantro
- ½ of a juiced lime
- Salt as needed
- Pepper as needed

Directions

1. Take a medium-sized bowl and add onion, tomato, avocados, bell pepper, lime juice and cilantro
2. Toss well
3. Season with pepper and salt
4. Serve chilled!

Nutritional Values per Serving

- Calories: 126
- Fat: 10g
- Carbohydrates: 10g
- Protein: 2.1g

Carrot Crisps

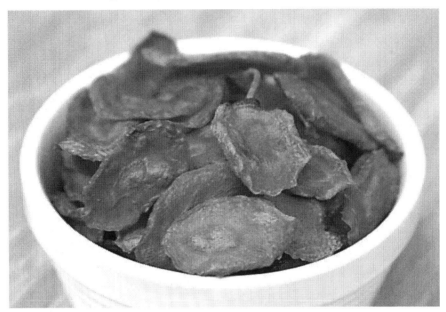

Serves: 4

Prep Time: 50 minutes

Cook Time: 10 minute

- 3 cups of carrots sliced paper thin
- 2 tablespoon of olive oil
- 2 teaspoon of ground cumin
- ½ a teaspoon of smoked paprika
- Pinch of salt

Directions

1. Pre-heat your oven to 215 degrees Fahrenheit
2. Slice up the carrots into paper-thin coin shapes
3. Add the slices to a bowl and toss well with spices and oil
4. Mix and lay them out on a baking sheet lined up with parchment paper

5. Sprinkle salt
6. Bake for 8-10 minutes and enjoy!

Nutritional Values per Serving

- Calories: 150
- Fat: 9g
- Carbohydrates: 15g
- Protein: 2g

Butternut Bisque of Coolness

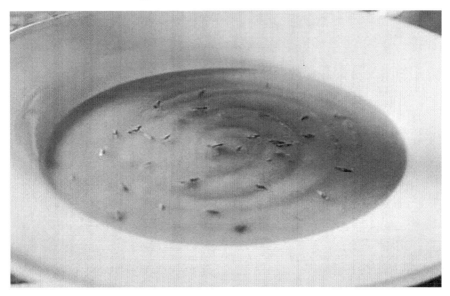

Serves: 4

Prep Time: 10 minutes

Cook Time: 70 minute

- 1 tablespoon of canola oil
- ½ a cup of diced onion
- ¾ cup of diced carrots
- 4 cups of peeled and cubed butternut squash
- 3 cups of vegetable stock
- Salt as needed
- Pepper as needed
- Ground nutmeg
- ½ a cup of cashew cream

Directions

1. Take a large sized pot and place it over medium-heat
2. Add oil and heat it up

3. Stir in onion and cook until tender
4. Add carrots and squash to your pot
5. Pour vegetable stock and season with pepper, salt, and nutmeg
6. Bring the mix to a boil and lower down the heat, simmer until the veggies are tender
7. Transfer to a food blender and puree
8. Stir in cashew cream and stir
9. Serve with a dash of nutmeg

Nutritional Values per Serving

- Calories: 127
- Fat: 5g
- Carbohydrates: 20g
- Protein: 3g

Slow Cooked Baked Potato

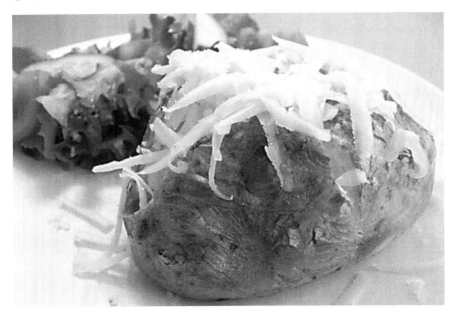

Serves: 4

Prep Time: 10 minutes

Cook Time: 4 hours 30 minutes

Ingredients

- 4 pieces of baking potatoes
- 1 tablespoon of extra virgin olive oil
- Kosher salt as needed
- 4 sheets of aluminum foil

Directions

1. Prick the potatoes with fork several times
2. Rub the potato with olive oil all over
3. Sprinkle salt
4. Place them tightly wrapped in your slow cooker and cook on HIGH for 4 and a ½ hour until tender
5. Serve and enjoy!

Nutritional Values per Serving

- Calories: 254
- Fat: 4g
- Carbohydrates: 51g
- Protein: 6g

Very Cute Cauliflower Salad

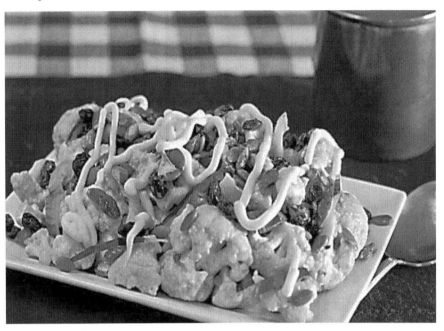

Serves: 2

Prep Time: 8 minutes

Cook Time: 0 minutes

Ingredients

- 1 head of cauliflower, broken up into bite-sized pieces
- 1 small sized onion chopped up
- 1/8 cup of extra virgin olive oil
- ¼ cup of apple cider vinegar
- ½ a teaspoon of sea salt
- ½ a teaspoon of black pepper
- ¼ cup of dried cranberries
- ¼ cup of pumpkin seeds

Directions

1. Wash up and break your cauliflower into bite-sized portions and add them to a bowl
2. Whisk oil, vinegar, salt and pepper in another bowl
3. Add pumpkin seeds, dried cranberries, and prepared dressing to your cauliflower
4. Add onion and toss well
5. Allow it to chill overnight
6. Serve and enjoy!

Nutritional Values per Serving

- Calories: 163
- Fat:11g
- Carbohydrates: 16g
- Protein: 3g

Very Cool and "Offbeat" Melon Soup

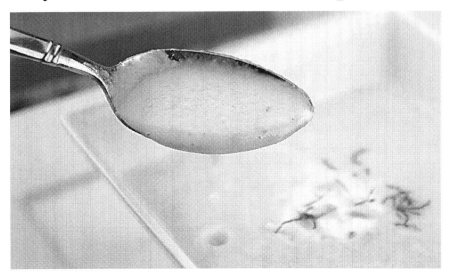

Serves: 4

Prep Time: 15 minutes

Cook Time: 0 minutes

Ingredients

- 4 cups of casaba melon, cubed and seeded
- ¾ cup of coconut milk
- Juice of 2 lime
- 1 tablespoon of freshly grated ginger
- 1 pinch of salt

Directions

1. Add the coconut milk, casaba melon, lime juice, salt and ginger to your food processor
2. Process it for about 1-2 minutes until the mixture has a soup-like texture
3. Enjoy!

Nutritional Values per Serving

- Calories: 134
- Fats: 9g
- Carbs:13g
- Protein:2g

Chapter 14: Dinner Recipes

Italian Kale Mix

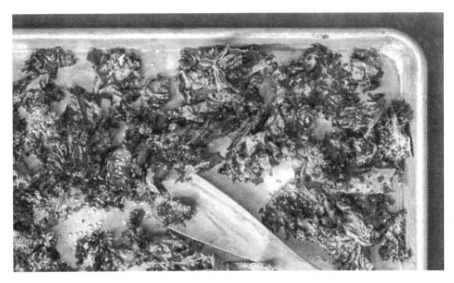

Serves: 4

Prep Time: 5 minutes

Cook Time: 15 minutes

Ingredients

- 1 bunch of kale with the stems removed and the leaves coarsely chopped
- 1 minced garlic cloves
- 1 tablespoon of olive oil
- 2 tablespoon of balsamic vinegar
- Salt as needed
- Pepper as needed

Directions

1. Take a large sized saucepan and place it over medium-high heat

2. Add kale and cook until the leaves wilt
3. Once the volume of kale has lowered to half, uncover the pan and stir in olive oil, vinegar, and garlic
4. Cook for 2 minutes more
5. Season with pepper and salt
6. Enjoy!

Nutritional Values per Serving

- Calories: 92
- Fat: 4g
- Carbohydrates: 12g
- Protein: 4g

Chilli Cold Thai Salad

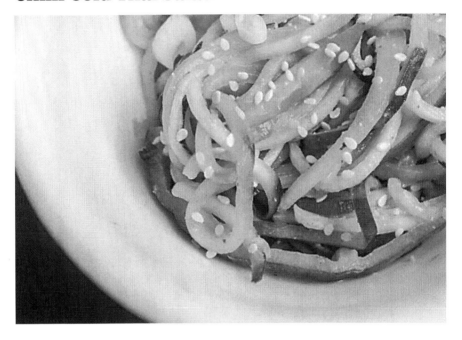

Prep Time: 25 minutes + 30 minutes chill time

Cooking Time: 0 minute

Serves: 2

Ingredients

- 2 small zucchini pieces
- 1 small cucumber
- 2 peeled and shredded carrots
- ½ a cup of mung bean sprouts
- ¼ cup chopped cashews
- ¼ cup chopped fresh cilantro
- ½ a cup of sunshine sauce

For Sauce

- ½ a cup of unsweetened sunflower seed butter

- ½ a cup of coconut milk
- 1 lime juiced
- 1 tablespoon of coconut aminos
- 1 minced garlic clove
- ½ a teaspoon of crushed red pepper flakes
- ½ a teaspoon of rice vinegar

Directions

1. Prepare the sauce by adding all of the listed ingredients in a small bowl and using it accordingly
2. Peel your zucchini using a regular peeler and make long slices using a julienne peeler
3. Keep peeling until all four sides are peeled
4. Repeat with all zucchini and cucumber
5. Add the noodles to a medium sized mixing bowl
6. Add shredded carrots, bean sprouts, chopped cashews, and cilantro
7. Chill for 30 minutes
8. Add a tablespoon of water to the Sunshine Sauce and tin it out
9. Pour it over your salad and garnish with a bit more cashews and cilantro
10. Enjoy!

Nutritional Values per Serving

- Protein: 4g
- Carbs: 19g
- Fats: 12g
- Calories: 187

Man's Best Friend Sweet Pepper Skillet

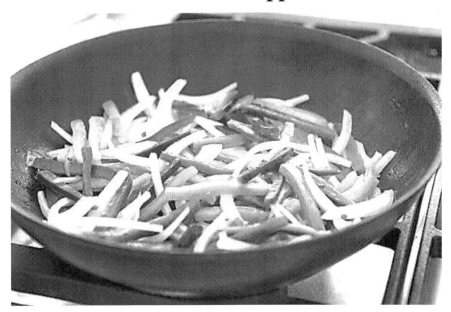

Serves: 4

Prep Time: 15 minutes

Cook Time: 10 minute

- 2 teaspoon of extra virgin olive oil
- 2 teaspoon of sesame oil
- 3 thinly sliced green bell peppers
- 1 chopped up yellow bell pepper
- 1 chopped up red bell peppers
- 1 chopped up red onion
- 2 teaspoon of minced garlic
- ¼ teaspoon of salt
- ¼ teaspoon of ground black pepper

Directions

1. Take a large sized skillet and place it over medium heat

2. Add olive oil and sesame oil, allow them to heat up
3. Add the peppers, red onion, garlic, pepper, and salt
4. Cook and stir for about 7-10 minutes until the peppers are cooked thoroughly
5. Enjoy!

<u>Nutritional Values per Serving</u>

- Calories: 109
- Fat: 1g
- Carbohydrates: 25g
- Protein: 1g

Indian Aloo Gobi Dish

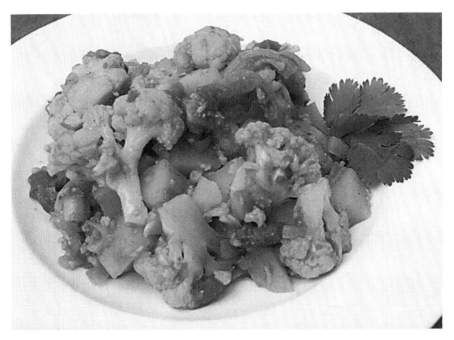

Serves: 2

Prep Time: 15 minutes

Cook Time: 20 minutes

Ingredients

- 1 tablespoon of vegetable oil
- 1 teaspoon of cumin seeds
- 1 teaspoon of minced garlic
- 1 teaspoon of ginger paste
- 2 medium-sized peeled and cubed potatoes
- ½ a teaspoon of ground turmeric
- ½ a teaspoon of paprika
- 1 teaspoon of ground cumin
- ½ a teaspoon of Garam masala
- Salt as needed
- 1 pound of cauliflower

- 1 teaspoon of chopped fresh cilantro

Directions

1. Take a medium-sized skillet and place it over medium heat
2. Add oil and stir in cumin seeds, ginger paste, and garlic
3. Cook for 1 minute until the garlic is browned up
4. Add potatoes and season with paprika, turmeric, Garam masala, salt and cumin
5. Cover and cook for 5-7 minutes more
6. Add cauliflower and cilantro to the pan
7. Lower down the heat and simmer for 10 minutes
8. Enjoy!

Nutritional Values per Serving

- Calories: 135
- Fat:4g
- Carbohydrates: 23g
- Protein: 4g

Strawberries and Balsamic Medley

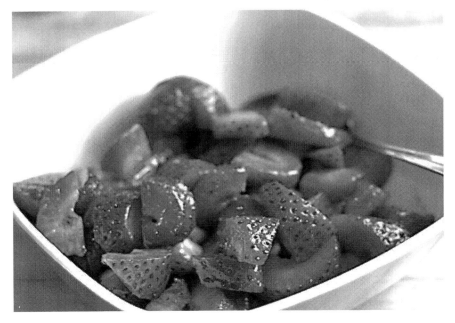

Serves: 6

Prep Time: 10 minutes

Cook Time: 0 minute

- 16 ounces of fresh strawberries, hulled, and large berries cut in half
- 2 tablespoon of balsamic vinegar
- 1 tablespoon of date paste
- ¼ teaspoon of freshly ground black pepper

Directions

1. Take a large sized bowl and add strawberries
2. Drizzle vinegar on top and mix with date paste
3. Stir well and combine
4. Sit for 1 hour and grind a bit of pepper
5. Serve!

Nutritional Values per Serving

- Calories: 200
- Fat: 18g
- Carbohydrates: 20g
- Protein: 3g

Grilled Potatoes

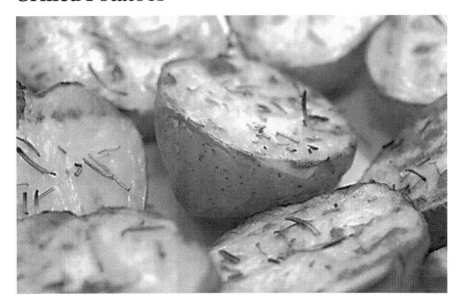

Serves: 4

Prep Time: 5 minutes

Cook Time: 22 minutes

Ingredients

- 2 large sized russet potatoes
- 2 tablespoon of olive oil
- Salt as needed
- Pepper as needed

Directions

1. Poke each of your potatoes and penetrate them with fork
2. Place your potatoes in your oven and cook on high power for about 5 minutes
3. Turn the potatoes about half way through while cooking
4. Slice up the potatoes in half and cook them for another 2 minutes on high power
5. Pre-heat your grill to medium heat

6. Brush up the top of your potato with olive oil and season with some pepper and salt
7. Cook on your grill for about 15-20 minutes, making sure to turn them once!
8. Serve!

Nutritional Values per Serving

- Calories: 203
- Fat: 7g
- Carbohydrates: 32g
- Protein: 4g

Highly Appreciable Pina Colada Coleslaw

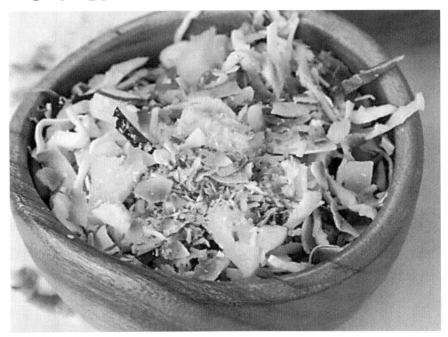

<u>**Serves:**</u> 5

<u>**Prep Time:**</u> **15 minutes**

<u>**Cook Time:**</u> **10 minute**

- 8 cups of shredded cabbage
- 1 cup of diced pineapple
- 1 cup of shredded coconut
- ½ a cup of coconut milk
- ½ a cup of pineapple juice
- 1 teaspoon of apple cider vinegar
- ¼ teaspoon of salt
- Sliced up almonds and macadamia nuts

<u>**Directions**</u>

1. Set your broiler on Low and take a baking sheet

2. Spread the coconut chips on your baking sheet and toast them under the broiler
3. Take them out and pour sliced cabbage in a bowl and add pineapple
4. For the dressing, add coconut milk, apple cider vinegar, pineapple juice, salt, and mix
5. Drizzle it over the cabbage mix
6. Add ½ a cup of your toasted coconut and mix
7. Chill and serve with an additional topping of almonds
8. Enjoy!

Nutritional Values per Serving

- Calories: 142
- Fat: 11g
- Carbohydrates: 9g
- Protein: 1g

Roasted Beets and Greens

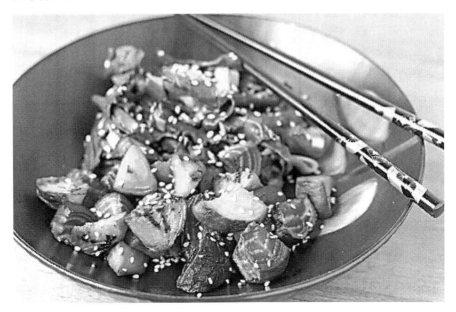

Serves: 4

Prep Time: 10 minutes

Cook Time: 30 minutes

Ingredients

- 1 bunch of beets with greens
- ¼ cup of divide olive oil
- 2 minced garlic cloves
- 2 tablespoon of chopped onion
- Salt as needed
- Pepper as needed
- 1 tablespoon of red wine vinegar

Directions

1. Pre-heat your oven to 350 degrees Fahrenheit
2. Wash the beets thoroughly

3. Remove the greens and rinse them separately, making sure to remove any stem

4. Keep them on the side

5. Place the beets in a small sized baking dish and toss with two tablespoons of olive oil until fully coated

6. Cover and bake the beets for 45-60 minutes in your oven

7. Once the beets are done, take a skillet over medium-low heat and pour two tablespoons of olive oil

8. Add garlic, onion and cook it for another minute

9. Tear up the beet greens into 2-3 inch pieces and add them to the skillet

10. Cook and keep stirring until the greens are soft and wilted

11. Season them with pepper and salt

12. Serve the green as they are

13. Serve the beets by seasoning them with some salt/pepper or red-wine vinegar

Nutritional Values per Serving

- Calories: 204
- Fat: 13g
- Carbohydrates: 18g
- Protein: 5.3g

Roasted Okra

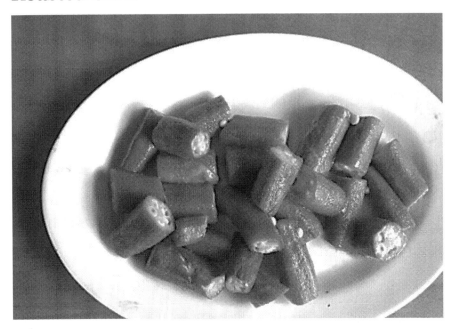

Serves: 2

Prep Time: 5 minutes

Cook Time: 15 minutes

Ingredients

- 18 fresh okra pods sliced up into 1/3 inch thick slices
- 1 tablespoon of olive oil
- 2 teaspoon of kosher salt
- 2 teaspoon of black pepper

Directions

1. Pre-heat your oven to 425 degrees Fahrenheit
2. Arrange the okra slices in one layer on a nice cookie sheet lined with foil
3. Drizzle some olive oil over them
4. Sprinkle some pepper and salt

5. Bake in your pre-heated oven for about 10-15 minutes
6. Serve hot

<u>Nutritional Values per Serving</u>

- Calories: 204
- Fat: 13g
- Carbohydrates: 18g
- Protein: 5.3g

Carrot Ribbons Rosemary Coconut Oil

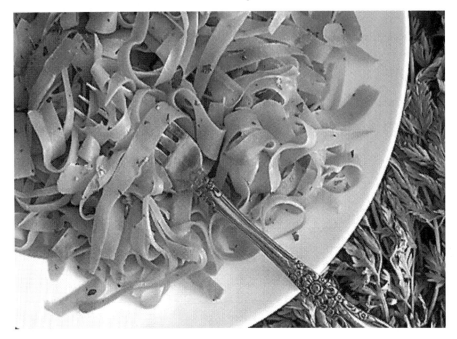

Serves: 2

Prep Time: 10 minutes

Cook Time: 3 minute

- 3-4 large straight carrots
- 1 tablespoon of coconut oil
- ½ a teaspoon of fresh rosemary minced up
- ½ a teaspoon of fresh minced parsley
- ¼ teaspoon of salt

Directions

1. Thoroughly wash your carrots and lay them on a counter
2. Use a vegetable peeler to peel the carrots and create ribbons
3. Keep repeating until all the carrots are used

4. Take a saucepan and place it over medium heat
5. Add enough water to fill it up and bring it to a boil
6. Add carrot in a metal colander and place it in your saucepan
7. Cover and steam for 3 minutes
8. Take a small bowl and add the rest of the ingredients
9. Add the steamed ribbons to the bowl and toss
10. Enjoy!

Nutritional Values per Serving

- Calories: 164
- Fat: 11g
- Carbohydrates: 16g
- Protein: 4g

Crispy Cabbage and Potatoes

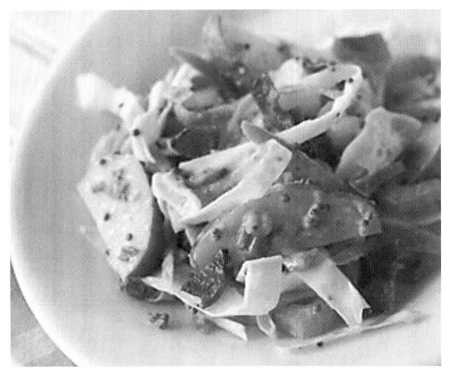

Serves: 4

Prep Time: 25 minutes

Cook Time: 40 minute

- ½ a cup of olive oil
- 4 thinly sliced carrots
- 1 thinly sliced onion
- 1 teaspoon of sea salt
- ½ a teaspoon of ground black pepper
- ½ a teaspoon of ground cumin
- ¼ teaspoon of ground turmeric
- ½ of a shredded cabbage head
- 5 peeled potatoes cut up into 1-inch cubes

Directions

1. Take a skillet and place it over medium heat
2. Add olive oil and heat it up
3. Add carrots, onion and cook them for 5 minutes
4. Stir in salt, cumin, pepper, turmeric, cabbage and cook for 15-20 minutes
5. Add potatoes
6. Cover and lower down the heat to medium-low
7. Cook for 20-30 minutes until the potatoes are tender

Nutritional Values per Serving

- Calories: 276
- Fat: 19g
- Carbohydrates: 13g
- Protein: 12g

Cool Fried Onions

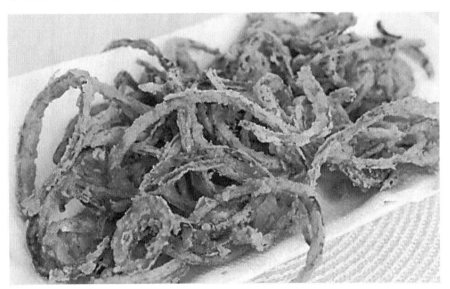

Serves: 12

Prep Time: 15 minutes

Cook Time: 20 minute

- 1 quart of olive oil
- 1 cup of almond flour
- 1 pinch of salt
- 1 pinch of ground black pepper
- 4 pieces of onions peeled and slice up into rings

Directions

1. Take a large sized deep skillet and heat up the oil to 365 degrees Fahrenheit
2. Take a medium-sized bowl and add flour, pepper, and salt
3. Dredge the onions in the mix until they are coated well
4. Deep fry the onions until they are golden brown
5. Drain them on paper towels

6. Enjoy!

Nutritional Values per Serving

- Calories: 421
- Fat: 6g
- Carbohydrates: 23g
- Protein: 9g

Heartwarming Cabbage Soup

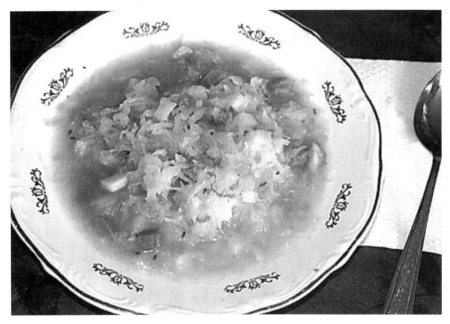

<u>Serves:</u> 8

<u>Prep Time:</u> 30 minutes

<u>Cook Time:</u> 45 minute

- 3 tablespoon of olive oil
- ½ of a chopped onion
- 2 chopped garlic cloves
- 2 quarts of water
- 1 teaspoon of salt
- ½ a teaspoon of black pepper
- ½ of a cabbage head (chopped and cored)
- 14 ounce of drained and diced tomatoes

Directions

1. Take a large sized stock pot and pour olive oil, heat it up over medium heat
2. Stir in garlic and onion once the oil is hot

3. Bring it to a boil
4. Stir in cabbage and simmer for 10 minutes
5. Stir in tomatoes and bring to a boil again
6. Simmer for 15-30 minutes
7. Keep stirring from time to time and serve!

Nutritional Values per Serving

- Calories: 92
- Fat: 5.2g
- Carbohydrates: 8.6g
- Protein: 1.5g

Majestic Heirloom Carrots

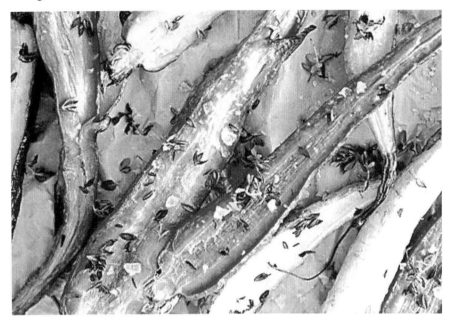

Serves: 3-4

Prep Time: 10 minutes

Cook Time: 45 minute

- 1 bunch of fine heirloom carrots
- 1 tablespoon of fresh thyme leaves
- ½ a tablespoon of coconut oil
- 1 tablespoon of date paste
- 1/8 cup of fresh squeezed orange juices
- 1/8 teaspoon of sea salt
- Salt as needed

Directions

1. Pre-heat your oven to 350 degrees Fahrenheit
2. Wash the carrots and discard green pieces

3. Take a small sized bowl and add coconut oil, orange juice, date paste and salt
4. Pour the mix over the carrot spread on a large sized baking sheet
5. Sprinkle thyme and roast for 45 minutes
6. Sprinkle salt and thyme on top and enjoy!

Nutritional Values per Serving

- Calories: 70
- Fat: 3g
- Carbohydrates: 11g
- Protein: 1g

Vegetable Fajitas

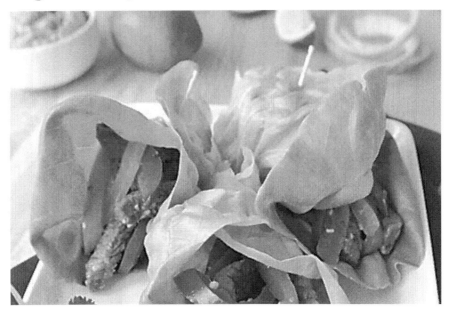

<u>**Serves:**</u> **4**

<u>**Prep Time:**</u> **30 minutes**

<u>**Cook Time:**</u> **20 minute**

- 2 teaspoon of olive oil
- 2 minced garlic cloves
- 2 sliced green bell peppers
- 2 sliced yellow bell pepper
- ½ of a sliced onion
- 1 cup of sliced mushrooms
- 3 chopped green onions
- Lemon pepper as needed

Directions

1. Take a large sized frying pan and place it over medium heat
2. Add olive oil and Saute garlic for 2 minutes

3. Stir in yellow and green bell peppers
4. Saute for 2 minutes
5. Stir in onion and Saute for another 2 minutes
6. Add green onions and mushrooms to the pan
7. Season with lemon pepper and stir
8. Cover and cook until the veggies are tender
9. Serve over beds of lettuce to make "Fajitas"

Nutritional Values per Serving

- Calories: 258
- Fat: 9g
- Carbohydrates: 35g
- Protein: 10g

Sweet Potato Noodle and Spinach Cashew

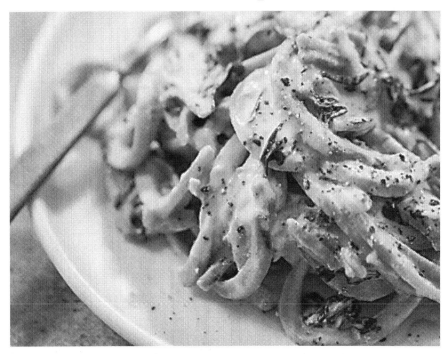

<u>**Serves:**</u> 4

<u>**Prep Time:**</u> **15 minutes**

<u>**Cook Time:**</u> **10 minute**

- 1 cup of cashews
- ¾ cup of water
- ½ a teaspoon of salt
- 1 clove of garlic
- 1 tablespoon of olive oil
- 4 large sized spiralized sweet potatoes
- 2 cups of baby spinach
- A handful of basil leaves
- Salt as needed
- Pepper as needed

- Olive oil for drizzling

Directions

1. Cover the cashews with water and soak for 2 hours
2. Drain them and add to your food processor
3. Add ¾ cup of water, garlic, and salt
4. Puree until the mixture is smooth
5. Take a large skillet and place it over high heat
6. Add sweet potatoes and toss well for 6-7 minutes
7. Remove the heat and add spinach
8. Add half of your herbs and half of your sauce
9. Season with salt and pepper
10. Drizzle olive oil and top with remaining fresh herbs
11. Serve!

Nutritional Values per Serving

- Calories: 448
- Fat: 17g
- Carbohydrates: 64g
- Protein: 12g

Mushroom and Tomato Spaghetti Squash

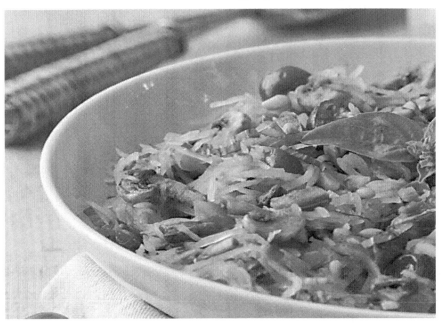

Serves: 4

Prep Time: 30 minutes

Cook Time: 10 minute

- 2 cooked spaghetti squash
- 2 cups of diced tomatoes
- 4 cloves of minced garlic
- 1/3 cup chopped onions
- ¼ cup of toasted pine nuts
- A handful of fresh basil
- 3 tablespoon of olive oil
- Kosher salt
- Black pepper as needed
- Pinch of red pepper flakes

Directions

1. Slice up your cooked spaghetti squash in half and remove the seeds and stringy bits
2. Shred it up using two forks
3. Take a large sauté pan and add oil, allow the oil to heat up
4. Add onion and mushroom and cook for 3-4 minutes
5. Add garlic and stir for 2 minute
6. Add tomatoes
7. Add cooked squash and toss well
8. Toss with fresh basil and toasted pine nuts
9. Season with kosher salt, pinch of red pepper flakes and enjoy!

Nutritional Values per Serving

- Calories: 325
- Fat: 10g
- Carbohydrates: 30g
- Protein: 10g

Avocado and Fennel Medley

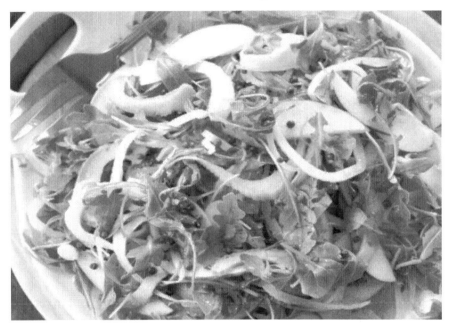

<u>**Serves:**</u> **4**

<u>**Prep Time:**</u> **10 minutes**

<u>**Cook Time:**</u> **0 minute**

- 3 thinly sliced fennel bulbs
- 1 peeled, cubed and pitted avocado
- 2 tablespoon of extra virgin olive oil
- 1 teaspoon of ground nutmeg
- Salt as needed

<u>Directions</u>

1. Take a salad bowl and add avocado, fennel
2. Stir in oil, nutmeg, salt and mix
3. Serve and enjoy!

Nutritional Values per Serving

- Calories: 130
- Fat: 8.4g
- Carbohydrates: 13.8g
- Protein: 2.4g

Stuffed Portobello Mushrooms

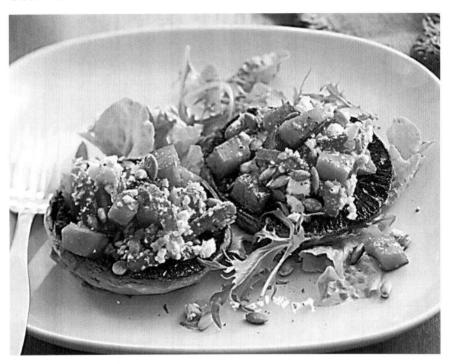

Serves: 4

Prep Time: 10 minutes

Cook Time: 15 minute

- 16 ounce of medium Portobello mushroom
- 1 small sized chopped onion
- 1 small sized red bell pepper chopped up
- 1 small sized stalk celery
- 2 minced garlic cloves
- ½ an inch of sliced up fresh ginger
- ½ a cup of pecans crushed up
- 1 tablespoon of olive oil
- Fresh ground black pepper

Directions

1. Preheat your oven to 350 degrees Fahrenheit
2. Line up a baking sheet with parchment paper
3. Pop up the stem of your mushroom and arrange the caps on your baking sheet
4. Chop up the stems and add them to a mixing bowl
5. Chop up the remaining veggies and add them to your bowl
6. Stir in pecans
7. Heat up a skillet and place it over medium heat and add oil
8. Allow the oil to heat up and add the bowl contents to your skillet
9. Saute for 4-5 minutes
10. Remove the heat and allow it to cool
11. Stir in black pepper
12. Spoon the mixture into your mushroom caps and bake for 15 minutes
13. Enjoy!

Nutritional Values per Serving

- Calories: 130
- Fat: 8.4g
- Carbohydrates: 13.8g
- Protein: 2.4g

Delightful Turmeric Soup

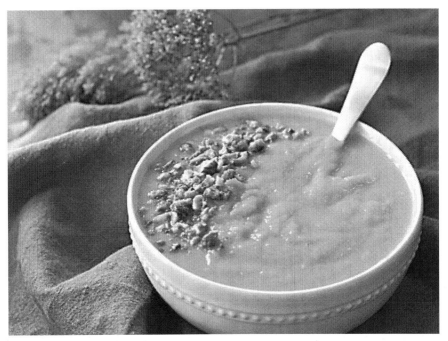

Prep Time: 5 minutes

Cooking Time: 25 minute

Serves: 4

Ingredients:

- 5 teaspoon of vegan stock
- 2 and a ½ cups of chopped carrots
- ½ an inch nub of fresh ginger
- 3.5 ounce of walnuts
- 1 teaspoon of turmeric
- ½ a teaspoon of cumin
- ½ a teaspoon of cinnamon
- 1 teaspoon of garlic powder
- 1 teaspoon of lemon juice

- 1 teaspoon of chipotle paste

Directions:

1. Add the listed ingredients to a stock pot and place it over medium-high heat
2. Simmer for 25 minutes
3. Blend the whole mixture using an immersion blender and enjoy!

Nutritional Values per Serving

- Calories: 207
- Fat: 4g
- Carbohydrates: 35g
- Protein: 10g

Chapter 15: The Epic Meal Plan

The following Meal Plan will help you to prepare yourself for the upcoming 30 days and plan what meal you are going to eat. Keep in mind that all of the recipes found in the meal plan are taken from the book.

You can easily alter the recipes according to your preferences and create your own meal plan!

If you feel that you require additional protein for your body, feel free to add plant-based protein powder in your food or juices or smoothies (some of the plant-based protein powder are pea protein powder, hemp protein powder, pumpkin protein powder, cranberry protein powder, and so on).

After each meal, I have included a short list of the required ingredients for the recipes, which will help you to shop for the meals ahead of time!

Bon Appetite!

Week 1 Meal Plan

Week 1	Breakfast	Lunch	Dinner
Day 1	Roasted Cauliflower Soup	Butternut Bisque of Coolness	Italian Kale Mix
Day 2	All-Star Baked Apple	Mushroom, Beet and Avocado Salad	Heartwarming Cabbage Soup
Day 3	Banana Bites	Another Green Smoothie	Man's Best Friend Sweet Pepper Skillet
Day 4	Roasted Cauliflower Soup	Butternut Bisque of Coolness	Italian Kale Mix
Day 5	All-Star Baked Apple	Mushroom, Beet and Avocado Salad	Heartwarming Cabbage Soup
Day 6	Banana Bites	Another Green Smoothie	Man's Best Friend Sweet Pepper Skillet
Day 7	Roasted Cauliflower Soup	Another Green Smoothie	Italian Kale Mix

Reference to Week 1 Shopping List

For Breakfast

Recipe 1: Roasted Cauliflower Soup

- 2 cauliflower head broken up into florets
- Olive oil cooking spray
- ¼ cup of olive oil
- 1 chopped up a large onion
- 4 cloves of chopped up garlic
- 6 cups of water
- Salt as needed
- Pepper as needed

Recipe 2: All-Star Bake Apple

- 1 piece of Fuji apple
- Raisins as needed
- Cinnamon as needed

Recipe 3: Banana Bites

- 4 teaspoon of cocoa powder (unsweetened)
- 4 teaspoon of toasted unsweetened coconut
- 2 sliced of small bananas

For Lunch

Recipe 1: Butternut Bisque of Coolness

- 1 tablespoon of canola oil
- ½ a cup of diced onion
- ¾ cup of diced carrots
- 4 cups of peeled and cubed butternut squash
- 3 cups of vegetable stock
- Salt as needed

- Pepper as needed
- Ground nutmeg
- ½ a cup of cashew cream

Recipe 2: Mushroom, Beet and Avocado Sauce

- 4 medium-sized Portobello mushroom caps
- ¼ cup of lemon juice
- 3 tablespoon of olive oil
- 1 small shallots finely chopped up
- 5 ounce of baby kale
- 8 ounce of precooked, chopped up beets
- 2 thinly sliced ripe avocados

Recipe 3: Another Green Smoothie

- 2 cups of coconut water
- 3.5 ounce of spinach
- 1 tablespoon of almond butter
- 2 small sized bananas
- 1 teaspoon of vanilla essence
- 1 tablespoon of hemp seeds
- 1 tablespoon of chia seeds

For Dinner

Recipe 1: Italian Kale Mix

- 1 bunch of kale with the stems removed and the leaves coarsely chopped
- 1 minced garlic cloves
- 1 tablespoon of olive oil
- 2 tablespoon of balsamic vinegar
- Salt as needed
- Pepper as needed

Recipe 2: Heartwarming Cabbage Soup

- 3 tablespoon of olive oil
- ½ of a chopped onion
- 2 chopped garlic cloves
- 2 quarts of water
- 1 teaspoon of salt
- ½ a teaspoon of black pepper
- ½ of a cabbage head (chopped and cored)
- 14 ounce of drained and diced tomatoes

Recipe 3: Man's Best Friend Sweet Pepper Skillet

- 2 teaspoon of extra virgin olive oil
- 2 teaspoon of sesame oil
- 3 thinly sliced green bell peppers
- 1 chopped up yellow bell pepper
- 1 chopped up red bell peppers
- 1 chopped up red onion
- 2 teaspoon of minced garlic
- ¼ teaspoon of salt
- ¼ teaspoon of ground black pepper

Week 2 Meal Plan

Week 2	Breakfast	Lunch	Dinner
Day 1	Easy Carrot Balls	Fancy Melon and Watercress Salad	Majestic Heirloom Potatoes
Day 2	Goodmorning Avocado Spread	Very Cool and "Offbeat" Melon Soup	Vegetable Fajitas
Day 3	Almond Berry Smoothie	Frozen Salad Bowl	Avocado and Fennel Medley
Day 4	Easy Carrot Balls	Fancy Melon and Watercress Salad	Majestic Heirloom Potatoes
Day 5	Goodmorning Avocado Spread	Very Cool and "Offbeat" Melon Soup	Vegetable Fajitas
Day 6	Almond Berry Smoothie	Frozen Salad Bowl	Avocado and Fennel Medley
Day 7	Almond Berry Smoothie	Fancy Melon and Watercress Salad	Majestic Heirloom Potatoes

Reference to Week 2 Shopping List

For Breakfast

Recipe 1: Easy Carrot Balls

- 6 pieces of pitted Medjool dates
- 1 finely grated carrot
- ¼ cup of raw walnuts
- ¼ cup of unsweetened finely shredded coconut
- 1 teaspoon of nutmeg
- 1/8 teaspoon of sea salt

Recipe 2: Good morning Avocado Spread

- 1 halved and pitted avocado
- 2 tablespoon of chopped fresh parsley
- 1 and a ½ teaspoon of extra virgin olive oil
- ½ a lemon juice
- ½ a teaspoon of salt
- ½ a teaspoon of ground black pepper
- ½ a teaspoon of onion powder
- ½ a teaspoon of garlic powder

Recipe 3: Almond Berry Smoothie

- 1 cup of frozen blueberries
- 1 piece of banana
- ½ a cup of almond milk
- 1 tablespoon of almond butter (Whole Foods Compliant Brand)
- Water as needed

For Lunch

Recipe 1: Fancy Melon Watercress Salad

- 3 tablespoon of fresh lime juice
- 1 teaspoon of date paste
- 1 teaspoon of minced fresh ginger root
- ¼ cup of vegetable oil
- 2 bunch of chopped up and trimmed watercress
- 2 and a ½ cups of cubed watermelon
- 2 and a ½ cups of cubed cantaloupe
- 1/3 cup of toasted and sliced almonds

Recipe 2: Very Cool and "Offbeat" Melon Soup

- 4 cups of casaba melon, cubed and seeded
- ¾ cup of coconut milk
- Juice of 2 lime
- 1 tablespoon of freshly grated ginger
- 1 pinch of salt

Recipe 3: Frozen Salad Bowl

- 2 cups of water
- ¼ cup of date paste
- 1 can of 20-ounces frozen orange juice concentrate (thawed)
- 1 can of 20-ounces frozen lemonade concentrate (thawed)
- 4 sliced up bananas
- 1 can of crushed pineapple (with juice)
- 1 pack of strawberries (thawed)

For Dinner

Recipe 1: Majestic Heirloom Carrot

- 1 bunch of fine heirloom carrots
- 1 tablespoon of fresh thyme leaves
- ½ a tablespoon of coconut oil
- 1 tablespoon of date paste

- 1/8 cup of fresh squeezed orange juices
- 1/8 teaspoon of sea salt
- Salt as needed

Recipe 2: Vegetable Fajitas

- 2 teaspoon of olive oil
- 2 minced garlic cloves
- 2 sliced green bell peppers
- 2 sliced yellow bell pepper
- ½ of a sliced onion
- 1 cup of sliced mushrooms
- 3 chopped green onions
- Lemon pepper as needed

Recipe 3: Avocado and Fennel Medley

- 3 thinly sliced fennel bulbs
- 1 peeled, cubed and pitted avocado
- 2 tablespoon of extra virgin olive oil
- 1 teaspoon of ground nutmeg
- Salt as needed

Week 3 Meal Plan

Week 3	Breakfast	Lunch	Dinner
Day 1	**Sunny Smoothie**	**Carrot Crisp**	**Strawberries and Balsamic Medley**
Day 2	**Green Smoothie**	**Apple and Kale Soup**	**Carrot Ribbons Rosemary Coconut Oil**
Day 3	**Plums From The Oven**	**Fresh Avocado and Cilantro Salad**	**Crispy Cabbage and Potatoes**
Day 4	**Sunny Smoothie**	**Carrot Crisp**	**Strawberries and Balsamic Medley**
Day 5	**Green Smoothie**	**Apple and Kale Soup**	**Carrot Ribbons Rosemary Coconut Oil**
Day 6	**Plums From The Oven**	**Fresh Avocado and Cilantro Salad**	**Crispy Cabbage and Potatoes**
Day 7	**Green Smoothie**	**Carrot Crisp**	**Strawberries and Balsamic Medley**

Reference to Week 3 Shopping List

For Breakfast

Recipe 1: Sunny Smoothie

- ½ of a frozen banana
- ½ a cup of fresh orange juice
- ¾ cup of frozen mango
- ¼ cup of water

Portion 2

- ½ of a frozen banana
- ¾ cup of frozen strawberries
- ½ a cup of water
- a few ice cubes

Recipe 2: Green Smoothie

- 1 cup of frozen mixed berries
- ½ a cup of baby spinach leaves
- 2 tablespoon of fresh orange juice
- 2 tablespoon of water
- 1 medium-sized ripe banana sliced up

Recipe 3: Plums From the Oven

- 4 pieces of plums, pitted and halved
- ½ a cup of orange juice
- 2 tablespoon of date paste
- ½ a teaspoon of ground cinnamon
- 1/8 teaspoon of ground nutmeg
- 1/8 teaspoon of cumin
- 1/8 teaspoon of cardamom
- ¼ cup of toasted and slivered almonds

For Lunch

Recipe 1: Carrot Crisps

- 3 cups of carrots sliced paper thin
- 2 tablespoon of olive oil
- 2 teaspoon of ground cumin
- ½ a teaspoon of smoked paprika
- Pinch of salt

Recipe 2: Apple and Kale Soup

- 8 walnut halves broken up into pieces
- 1 finely chopped up onion
- 2 coarsely grated carrots
- 2 unpeeled but finely chopped up red apples
- 1 tablespoon of cider vinegar
- 2 cups of reduced salt vegetable stock
- 7 ounce of roughly chopped kale
- 1 ounce of dried apple crisps

Recipe 3: Fresh Avocado and Cilantro Salad

- 2 avocados – peeled, pitted and diced
- 1 chopped up a sweet onion
- 1 green bell pepper (chopped up)
- 1 large sized chopped up a ripe tomato
- ¼ cup of chopped up fresh cilantro
- ½ of a juiced lime
- Salt as needed
- Pepper as needed

For Dinner

Recipe 1: Strawberries and Balsamic Medley

- 16 ounce of fresh strawberries hulled and large berries cut in half

- 2 tablespoon of balsamic vinegar
- 1 tablespoon of date paste
- ¼ teaspoon of freshly ground black pepper

Recipe 2: Carrot Ribbons Rosemary Coconut Oil

- 3-4 large straight carrots
- 1 tablespoon of coconut oil
- ½ a teaspoon of fresh rosemary minced up
- ½ a teaspoon of fresh minced parsley
- ¼ teaspoon of salt

Recipe 3: Crispy Cabbage and Potatoes

- ½ a cup of olive oil
- 4 thinly sliced carrots
- 1 thinly sliced onion
- 1 teaspoon of sea salt
- ½ a teaspoon of ground black pepper
- ½ a teaspoon of ground cumin
- ¼ teaspoon of ground turmeric
- ½ of a shredded cabbage head
- 5 peeled potatoes cut up into 1-inch cubes

Week 4 Meal Plan

Week 4	Breakfast	Lunch	Dinner
Day 1	Fantastic Almond "Vegan" Butter Balls	Butternut Bisque and Cilantro Salad	Cool Fried Onion
Day 2	Sweet Potato Noodle and Spinach Cashew	Grilled Guacamole Avocado	Majestic Heirloom Carrot
Day 3	Fried Apples	Extremely Fresh Pineapple Salsa	Roasted Okra
Day 4	Fantastic Almond "Vegan" Butter Balls	Butternut Bisque and Cilantro Salad	Cool Fried Onion
Day 5	Sweet Potato Noodle and Spinach Cashew	Grilled Guacamole Avocado	Majestic Heirloom Carrot
Day 6	Fried Apples	Extremely Fresh Pineapple Salsa	Roasted Okra
Day 7	Fantastic Almond "Vegan" Butter Balls	Butternut Bisque and Cilantro Salad	Cool Fried Onion

Reference to Week 4 Shopping List

For Breakfast

Recipe 1: Fantastic Almond "Vegan" Butter Balls

- 12 pieces of diced and pitted dates
- 1/3 cup of unsweetened shredded coconut
- 2 and a ½ tablespoon of almond butter

Recipe 2: Sweet Potato Noodle and Spinach Cashew

- 1 cup of cashews
- ¾ cup of water
- ½ a teaspoon of salt
- 1 clove of garlic
- 1 tablespoon of olive oil
- 4 large sized spiralized sweet potatoes
- 2 cups of baby spinach
- A handful of basil leaves
- Salt as needed
- Pepper as needed
- Olive oil for drizzling

Recipe 3: Fried Apples

- ½ a cup of coconut oil
- ¼ cup of date paste
- 2 tablespoon of ground cinnamon
- 4 pieces of Granny Smith Apples, peeled, sliced and cored

For Lunch

Recipe 1: Butternut Bisque and Cilantro Salad

- 1 tablespoon of canola oil

- ½ a cup of diced onion
- ¾ cup of diced carrots
- 4 cups of peeled and cubed butternut squash
- 3 cups of vegetable stock
- Salt as needed
- Pepper as needed
- Ground nutmeg
- ½ a cup of cashew cream

Recipe 2: Grilled Guacamole Avocado

- 5 whole pieces of avocados
- ¼ cup of diced red onion
- 1 whole jalapeno
- 2 cloves of garlic
- ¼ teaspoon of cumin
- ½ a teaspoon of smoked paprika
- ¼ teaspoon of salt
- ¼ teaspoon of black pepper
- ½ of a whole lime

Recipe 3: Extremely Fresh Pineapple Salsa

- ½ of pineapple cut up into small diced
- 2 teaspoon of chopped fine jalapeno
- 2 thinly sliced green onion
- 1 teaspoon of ground cumin
- 2 tablespoon of freshly squeezed lime juice
- ¼ cup of cilantro chopped up
- Salt as needed
- Pepper as needed

For Dinner

Recipe 1: Cool Fried Onions

- 1 quart of olive oil
- 1 cup of almond flour
- 1 pinch of salt
- 1 pinch of ground black pepper
- 4 pieces of onions peeled and slice up into rings

Recipe 2: Majestic Heirloom Carrots

- 1 bunch of fine heirloom carrots
- 1 tablespoon of fresh thyme leaves
- ½ a tablespoon of coconut oil
- 1 tablespoon of date paste
- 1/8 cup of fresh squeezed orange juices
- 1/8 teaspoon of sea salt
- Salt as needed

Recipe 3: Roasted Okra

- 18 fresh okra pods sliced up into 1/3 inch thick slices
- 1 tablespoon of olive oil
- 2 teaspoon of kosher salt
- 2 teaspoon of black pepper

Conclusion

I would like to thank you for purchasing the book and taking the time for going through the book as well.

I hope this book has been helpful and you found the information contained within the pages useful!

Keep in mind that you are not only limited to the recipes provided in this book! Just go ahead and continue exploring until you create your very own culinary masterpiece!

Stay healthy and stay safe!

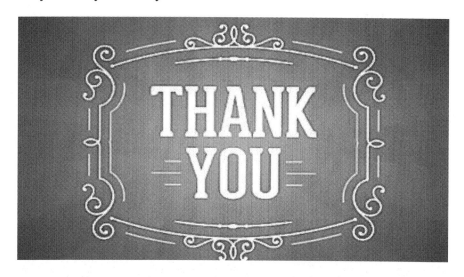

Made in the USA
Middletown, DE
19 April 2018